SHARED GOVERNANCE

*A Practical Approach to Transform
Professional Nursing Practice*

Second Edition

DIANA SWIHART,

PhD, DMin, MSN, CS, RN-BC

Foreword by **TIM PORTER-O'GRADY,**
DM, EdD, ScD(h), APRN, FAAN

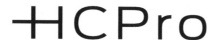

Shared Governance: A Practical Approach to Transform Professional Nursing Practice, Second Edition, is published by HCPro, Inc.

HCPro, Inc., provides information resources for the healthcare industry.

HCPro, Inc., is not affiliated in any way with The Joint Commission, which owns the JCAHO and Joint Commission trademarks. MAGNET™, MAGNET RECOGNITION PROGRAM®, and ANCC MAGNET RECOGNITION® are trademarks of the American Nurses Credentialing Center (ANCC). The products and services of HCPro, Inc., and The Greeley Company are neither sponsored nor endorsed by the ANCC. The acronym MRP is not a trademark of HCPro or its parent corporation.

Diana Swihart, PhD, DMin, MSN, CS, RN-BC, Author
Rebecca Hendren, Senior Managing Editor
Emily Sheahan, Group Publisher
Mike Mirabello, Senior Graphic Artist
Matt Sharpe, Production Supervisor
Shane Katz, Art Director
Jean St. Pierre, Senior Director of Operations

Arrangements can be made for quantity discounts. For more information, contact:

HCPro, Inc.
75 Sylvan Street, Suite A-101
Danvers, MA 01923
Telephone: 800/650-6787 or 781/639-1872
Fax: 781/639-7857
E-mail: *customerservice@hcpro.com*

Visit HCPro online at: *www.hcpro.com* and *www.hcmarketplace.com*

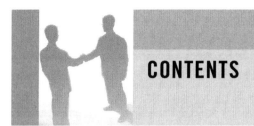

CONTENTS

CONTENTS

CONTENTS

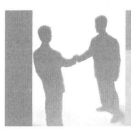

LIST OF FIGURES AND TOOLS TO HELP BUILD AND MEASURE SHARED GOVERNANCE

The following figures are included in the book:

The following tools and resources relate to information contained in these chapters. The appendixes are available for download at *www.hcpro.com/downloads/9581*.

                     SHARED GOVERNANCE, SECOND EDITION

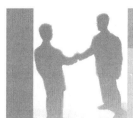

DEDICATION

This work is dedicated to those courageous and giving nurses who continue to teach me about the extraordinary realities of lived shared governance. These profound heroes and heroines exemplify professional nursing at its best through their passion, integrity, and commitment to excellence at every opportunity of service. Thank you.

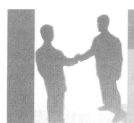

ABOUT THE AUTHOR

Diana Swihart, PhD, DMin, MSN, CS, RN-BC

Diana Swihart, PhD, DMin, MSN, CS, RN-BC, enjoys many roles in her professional career, practicing in widely diverse clinical and nonclinical settings. She is currently a regional nurse at the Denver Office of Clinical Consultation and Compliance, Veterans Health Administration. An author, speaker, researcher, educator, mentor, and consultant, she holds graduate degrees in nursing and leadership and doctorates in theology and ministry. She provided operational leadership for the shared governance processes for the Bay Pines (FL) VA Healthcare System and served as a liaison to help facilitate the application of evidence-based practice and nursing research.

She is a member of Sigma Theta Tau International, the Nurses Organization of Veterans Affairs, the Veterans Educators Integrated Network, and several professional advisory boards. She has published and spoken on a number of topics related to nursing, shared governance, competency assessment, continuing nursing education, nursing and servant leadership, the American Nurses Credentialing Center (ANCC) Magnet Recognition Program®, professional nurse development, building effective preceptorships, and evidence-based practice in clinical settings locally, nationally, and internationally. She published the first edition of *Shared Governance: A Practical Guide for Reshaping Professional Nursing Practice* in 2006. She served as an ANCC Magnet Recognition Program® appraiser for six years and as the treasurer for the National Nursing Staff Development Organization for four years. She currently serves as a commissioner on ANCC's Commission on Accreditation.

Dr. Swihart believes deeply in partnerships in healing and professional practice. Her training and multi-dimensional experiences give her a broad and balanced perspective of nursing that influences and colors all she does as she creatively challenges and encourages others in professional practice and environments of care.

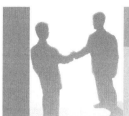

ACKNOWLEDGMENTS

Every work, regardless of scope and size, is completed only with the help and inspiration of others. My sincere thanks go to my beloved husband for his support and encouragement, his unwavering belief in me. I also want to thank my devoted son, who lent his own writing skills and gifts to the earlier reading and critiquing of the manuscript, helping me write in a way that would be more comfortable and interesting for readers.

I would also like to acknowledge those many other nurses and patients, speakers and teachers, and colleagues and friends who have contributed their ideas and thoughts through countless classes, seminars, lectures, and discussions I have experienced over the years. I write from their influence and want to recognize their contributions as well. Though their names are too numerous to list, many others can be found in this work and in the extended bibliography. To each and every one of you, thank you.

Finally, I would like to thank two innovative and courageous leaders in nursing today who have most transformed my own thinking about shared governance: Dr. Robert Hess, a friend and colleague who taught me to measure shared governance and how to see more clearly the potential for nurses to truly lead change and advance healthcare on every level; and Dr. Tim Porter-O'Grady, whose work first drew me to the study of shared governance. After studying more than 180 articles, videos, and books, my ideas and writing most strongly reflect Dr. Porter-O'Grady's influence. For this reason, I am particularly pleased that he has again written the foreword for what I hope to be another valuable addition to your own journey in helping reshape and transform professional nursing practice for this and the next generation.

Diana Swihart, PhD, DMin, MSN, CS, RN-BC
April 2011

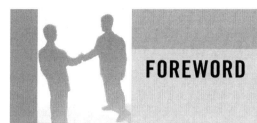

FOREWORD

The concept of shared governance continues to be a centerpiece of developing the collaborative environment for patient care. It continues to reflect the need to engage and empower people, and is the centerpiece of shared governance. Shared governance has been associated with good management for some 60 years. It seems to many that such concepts are new and innovative simply because so few leaders actually implement these concepts into the exercise of their own management. The prevailing model for management has historically been one that represents parent-child relationships, because it is the predominant model of leadership that most people can identify in the absence of real leadership education.

In nursing, much of management represents a parental and maternal influence that extends into the staff management interaction at every level of nursing practice. From the orientation program to policy, procedure, protocols, and practices, the nurse is constantly reminded of how much his or her life is scripted and controlled by external parameters and directives. It is no wonder that, given enough time, most nurses lose interest in controlling their own practice and influencing the practice lives of others. Ultimately, a nurse's locus of control becomes so narrow that he or she ceases to do anything but the most functional and routine activities and quickly becomes addicted to the predictable and ritualistic activities of nursing.

It is a challenge to get nurses out of their rut and fully engage them in their practice lives. Even when it is clearly in the best interest of the nurse to become more fully involved, the vagaries of work, the demands of patient care, and any other excuse becomes the barrier to fully engaging with those things that are necessary to advance and change practice. The leaders, for their part, have created such a vertical orientation and relationship that staff ultimately feel as though anything significant, important, or valuable can only be done by managers or by management mandate. They feel that any effort on the part of the staff infringes on their time and therefore is not legitimate. In this age of reform and interdisciplinary integration around an evidence-driven patient care model, the engaged and mature partnership role of the nurse is the essential centerpiece.

Shared governance reflects a completely different mental model for relationship and for leadership within and between disciplines. It recognizes that nursing as a profession coordinates, integrates, and facilitates the interface between the disciplines and around the patient. In fact, shared governance is predominantly about building a particular infrastructure or framework for building an effective interprofessional interaction between nursing and its care partners. It reorients the decision-making construct to require a broader distribution of decisions across the professions and allocates decisions based on accountability and role contributions to the collective work of patient care. This reconfiguration of the health system is intended to define staff-based decisions, accountability, roles, and ownership of all clinical staff in those activities that directly affect the care of the patient.

Success with shared governance requires a powerful reorientation of the organization. It requires leadership to understand that a significant retooling of leadership capacity and skill is required to successfully implement shared governance and sustain it as a way of life in the professional organization. Implementing shared governance means retraining managers, engaging staff, reallocating accountability, and building a truly staff-driven model of decision and action. Because behavior cannot be changed or sustained without a supporting infrastructure, it means redesigning and structuring the organization to eliminate rewards for passive behavior and enumerating and inculcating rewards for engagement within the very fabric of the organization.

Staff-driven decision-making is a strong indicator of excellence. It is no surprise that the American Nurses Credentialing Center Magnet Recognition Program® bases its major themes in a way that reflects the values and system of shared governance and staff-based accountability. Also, the work is not easy, and it cannot be done overnight. It means building an entire new culture that clearly and unambiguously reflects the characteristics of a truly collaborative, professional organization. From the highest levels of organizational leadership to the patient relationship, there must be strong evidence of practice driving the organization's work. In all professions, power is grounded in practice. Excellence in practice can only be obtained and sustained if the practitioners hold and exercise the power that only practice can drive in achieving excellence and satisfaction. Without it, the power to influence, change, challenge, and "push the walls" toward innovation and creativity is simply vacated, and others end up playing that role, whether their doing so is legitimate or not.

Sharon Finnigan and I wrote the first definitive book on shared governance in 1985. Although we and others have continued to add to that body of knowledge over the years, no substantial foundational text on implementing the basics of an effective shared governance system has been forthcoming since that time, until this current work (written first in 2006, now expanded in 2011). Here, the author has clearly enumerated the foundations of shared governance and the practical elements necessary to construct a shared governance structure (including the interdisciplinary requisites) and to make it successful. This is perhaps one of the clearest explications of the principles, design, and processes associated with a viable and successful shared governance model that exists in the literature today.

If the reader carefully works through this text and thoughtfully reasons and applies the principles set out herein, he or she can advance the opportunity to create a successful approach to broad-based shared governance. Each stage of development, every design element, components of the decision process, and evaluation of effectiveness outlined here provides the tools necessary to make implementation successful. Although the work will be focused and sometimes difficult, the rewards have proven to be substantial to those who have been willing to risk the effort and initiate the dynamic of creating a truly professional patient-centered organization. There is no greater indicator of a viable and sustainable potential for nurses and the clinical team—as well as those we serve—than a fully empowered and engaged professional community that creates the foundations and conditions for excellence for the foreseeable future.

Tim Porter-O'Grady, DM, EdD, ScD(h), APRN, FAAN
Senior Partner, Tim Porter-O'Grady Associates, Inc.
Atlanta, GA

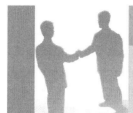

PREFACE

Why a second edition of a shared governance book devoted to the "how to" approach to implementing this particular model? When the first edition was written, it was specifically to fill an identified need. As a new American Nurses Credentialing Center Magnet Recognition Program® (MRP) director, I was asked to design a shared governance structure for a growing multifacility healthcare system as part of its journey to excellence and MRP designation. Direct-care nurses and leaders described the concept as "shared decision-making" or "shared leadership" without being able to identify specifics of what that might look like as part of shared governance in practice or how to get there.

As I investigated how best to proceed, I found that even the most learned experts and consultants seemed to disagree on what shared governance was, much less how to apply it to the nursing meso- and micro-systems within the organization. Yet, nurse leaders such as Dr. Tim Porter-O'Grady had been developing and teaching the benefits and structures of shared governance for many years, while his friend and colleague Dr. Robert Hess had designed and validated instruments to measure it.

So why was shared governance not part of the lived experience of professional nurses at the point of service?

- Leaders believed shared governance was necessary and possible

- Direct-care nurses believed it was necessary but not possible

Therefore, in beginning the work in my own organization and carefully considering the evidence, I found that the theory, concept, and constructs for shared governance were all sound. The key lay in defining, describing, and applying them in practice settings. To do this, direct-care nurses needed clearly delineated guidance, templates, and tools.

Since that first publication, I have received a plethora of ideas, descriptions of repeated challenges across diverse organizations (e.g., nurses holding to legacy systems; insistence on micromanagement of professional nurses around practice, quality, and competency; leaders who manage but do not lead; direct-care nurses who disengage or even sabotage the efforts of engaged nurses at all levels; lack of resources and/or commitment to sustained shared governance), and contributions of best practices from nurses who work in organizations where shared governance is the lived experience—the business-as-usual approach to professional nursing practice in partnership with interprofessional and interdisciplinary team members.

I have been amazed and humbled at how well the first edition was received and the willingness of readers to share their thoughts, concerns, and recommendations for improving it as more organizations are formally devoting funds and other resources to shared governance. This second edition retains everything readers need from the first edition but with more clarity in defining terms, describing processes, and advancing professional nursing practice. It also contains suggestions for building unit-level councils and nursing governance councils in step-by-step format with tools and information addressing every need identified by direct-care nurses and nurse leaders over the past five years. Additionally, this work includes important information regarding the future of nursing (Institute of Medicine, 2011) and the critical need for nurses to engage in shared governance at the point of service to more successfully participate in building that future.

Diana Swihart, PhD, DMin, MSN, CS, RN-BC
June 2011

CONTINUING EDUCATION CREDITS AVAILABLE

Continuing education credits are available for this book for two years from date of purchase.

For more information about credits available, and to take the continuing education exam, please see the Nursing Education Instructional Guide found with the downloadable resources at *www.hcpro.com/downloads/9581*.

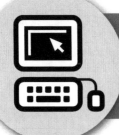 **DOWNLOAD YOUR MATERIALS NOW**

Readers of *Shared Governance: A Practical Approach to Transform Professional Nursing Practice*, Second Edition, can download the book's tools and templates at the HCPro Web address below. You will find figures from the book as well as all 35 bonus appendixes. The files are easily customized so you can adapt and use them at your facility today.

The continuing education quiz is also included with the downloadable resources. Find it within the Nursing Education Instructional Guide.

Find the tools online at:

www.hcpro.com/downloads/9581

HCPro

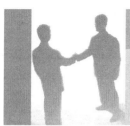

INTRODUCTION: THE CONSTRUCT OF SHARED GOVERNANCE

<table>
</table>

LEARNING OBJECTIVES

After reading this chapter, the participant should be able to:

- Define the four primary principles of shared governance: partnership, equity, accountability, and ownership

- Compare two professional nursing practice models

Nursing is the protection, promotion, and optimization of health and abilities, prevention of illness and injury, alleviation of suffering through the diagnosis and treatment of human response, and advocacy in the care of individuals, families, communities, and populations.

– American Nurses Association (2003)

The increasing criticality of the professional nurse shortage is a recurrent and dangerous theme in healthcare. A growing number of institutions are reexamining shared governance—a concept introduced into healthcare organizations in the 1970s—as an evidence-based method to curb the damaging effects of the shortage (e.g., negative patient outcomes, high cost of agency staff, and RN sign-on bonuses). This book takes some of the guesswork out of the various structures and processes behind shared governance and provides strategies, case examples, and best practices to make the daily operations of shared governance meaningful and successful. It also explores the relationship between shared governance and the American Nurses Credentialing Center (ANCC) Magnet Recognition Program® (MRP), outlining the MRP expectations for shared governance practices.

What Is Shared Governance?

> Before it can be solved, a problem must be clearly defined.
>
> *– William Feather*

Shared governance has been referred to as a concept, a construct, a model, a system, a philosophy, and even as a movement. It is most often called shared decision-making and/or shared leadership in many organizations that have implemented it. Before going any further, then, an operational definition is needed to clarify this work and address the research and applications to practice we find in shared governance.

> *Shared governance* is an innovative organizational management model; it is the <u>structure</u> for the <u>process</u> of shared decision-making and <u>outcomes</u> of shared leadership.

Because shared governance reflects the mission, vision, and values of those who embrace it, it appears to be a fluid presence in each environment and practice setting. In 1975, Dr. Luther Christman, a highly honored but controversial leader and provocative advocate for nursing (Pittman, 2006), spoke about an autonomous nursing organization at the American Nurses Association convention in Atlantic City, NJ. Other great nurses caught his vision and continue to build nursing as a profession through shared governance, such as Dr. Tim Porter-O'Grady and Dr. Robert Hess (see expanded bibliography, which for space reasons is included only online with the rest of the downloadable resources).

The *Random House Unabridged Dictionary* defines the verb *govern* as to exercise a directing or restraining influence over; guide: *the motives governing a decision*; to have predominating influence. Building on that context, Hess' research in measuring shared governance developed and validated an 86-item instrument specifically designed to assess the six domains of shared governance in an organization and in the profession of nursing related to control, influence, authority, participation, access, and ability. Most instruments measure characteristics and some outcomes related to shared governance. However, the Index for Professional Governance and the Index for Professional Nursing Governance have been researched and used to measure progress in developing and/or establishing shared governance in growing numbers of organizations.

See Chapter 6 for further details on the Index for Professional Governance and the Index for Professional Nursing Governance. You can find both these documents with the rest of the appendixes on the downloadable resources page at *www.hcpro.com/downloads/9581*. Look for App1 and App2 in the list of resources. In addition, see the expanded bibliography for more details on this topic.

> STRUCTURE: shared governance
> PROCESS: shared decision-making
> OUTCOME: shared leadership

The management process model of shared governance, *shared decision-making*, is based on the principles of partnership, equity, accountability, and ownership at the point of service. It empowers all members of the healthcare workforce to have a voice in decision-making. This facilitates diverse and creative input to advance the business and healthcare missions of the organization. In essence, this makes every employee feel like he or she is "part manager" with a personal stake in the success of the organization, which leads to:

+ Longevity of employment

+ Increased employee satisfaction

+ Better safety and healthcare

+ Greater patient satisfaction

+ Shorter lengths of stay

Those who are happy in their jobs take greater ownership of their decisions and are more vested in patient outcomes. Employees, patients, the organization, and the surrounding communities benefit from shared governance.

In effective shared governance, decision-making must be shared at the point of service to allow cost-effective service delivery and nurse empowerment. This requires a decentralized management structure. Employee partnership, equity, accountability, and ownership occur at the point of service (e.g., on the patient care units) where at least 90% of the decisions need to be made. The locus of control in the professional practice environment shifts to practitioners in matters of practice, quality, and competence. Only 10% of the decisions at the unit level belong to management (Porter-O'Grady & Hitchings, 2005).

Partnerships

Partnership links healthcare providers and patients along all points in the system; it is a collaborative relationship among all stakeholders and nursing required for professional empowerment. Partnership is essential to building relationships, involves all staff members in decisions and processes, implies that each member has a key role in fulfilling the mission and purpose of the organization, and is critical to the effectiveness of the healthcare system (Porter-O'Grady & Hitchings, 2005).

Equity

Equity is the best method for integrating staff roles and relationships into structures and processes to achieve positive patient outcomes. Equity maintains a focus on services, patients, and staff; is the foundation and measure of value; and says that no role is more important than another. Although equity does *not* equal equality in terms of scope of practice, knowledge, authority, or responsibility, it does mean that each team member is essential in providing safe and effective care (Porter-O'Grady & Hitchings, 2005; Porter-O'Grady, Hawkins, & Parker, 1997).

Accountability

Accountability is a willingness to invest in decision-making and express ownership in those decisions. Accountability is the core of shared governance. It is often used interchangeably with responsibility and allows evaluation of role performance. It facilitates partnerships for sharing decisions and is secured in the roles by staff producing positive outcomes (Porter-O'Grady & Hitchings, 2005). Figure 1.1 shows characteristics of accountability and responsibility.

Figure 1.1 — CHARACTERISTICS OF ACCOUNTABILITY AND RESPONSIBILITY

Accountability	Responsibility
Defined by outcomes	Defined by functions
Self-described	Delegated
Embedded in roles	Specific tasks/routines dictated
Dependent on partnerships	Isolative
Shares evaluation	Supervisor evaluation
Contributions-driven value	Tasks-driven value

Adapted from Porter-O'Grady and Hitchings (2005).

 SHARED GOVERNANCE, SECOND EDITION

Ownership

Ownership is recognition and acceptance of the importance of everyone's work and that an organization's success is bound to how well individual staff members perform their jobs. Ownership designates where work is done and by whom to enable participation of all team members. It requires a commitment by each staff member for what is to be contributed, establishes a level of authority with an obligation to own what is done, and includes participation in devising purposes for the work (Koloroutis, 2004; Page, 2004; Porter-O'Grady & Hitchings, 2005). Shared governance activities may include participatory scheduling, joint staffing decisions, and/or shared unit responsibilities (e.g., every RN is trained to be "in charge" of his or her unit or area and shares that role with other professional team members, perhaps on a rotating schedule) to achieve the best patient care outcomes.

The old centralized management structures for command and control are ineffective for today's healthcare market, frequently inhibiting effective change and growth within the organization and limiting future market possibilities in recruitment and retention of qualified nurses. Summative, hierarchical decision-making creates barriers to employee autonomy and empowerment. It can undermine service and quality of care. Today's patients are no longer satisfied with directive care. They, too, want partnership, equity, accountability, and mutual ownership in their own healthcare decisions and those of their family members (Institute of Medicine, 2011).

History and Development of Shared Governance

The concepts of shared governance and shared decision-making are not new ones. Philosophy, education, religion, politics, business and management, and healthcare have all benefited from a variety of shared governance process models implemented in many diverse and creative ways across generations and cultures.

- Socrates (470–399 BC), an ancient Greek philosopher, integrated shared governance concepts into his philosophies of education. The Socratic Method (answering a question with a question) calls for the teacher to facilitate the student's autonomous learning as the teacher guides him or her through a series of questions. The Socratic Method encourages students to use reason rather than appeal to authority.

- The government model for the United States was established on the concepts of shared governance— "of the people, by the people, for the people" (from Lincoln's *Gettysburg Address*, 1863)—wherein the very citizenry is directly responsible for the government on both state and federal levels. Political variations of this model of shared governance can also be seen in the European Union and the United Nations, where individual countries share in the decision-making on joint international matters.

+ Eventually, shared governance found its way into the business and management literature (Laschinger, 1996; O'May & Buchan, 1999; Peters & Waterman, 1982). Organizations began to design formal structures and relationships around their leaders and employees. Positive outcomes emphasized movement from point of service outward. This differed from the more traditional, hierarchical method of moving from the organization downward approach previously used.

+ In the late 1970s and early '80s, shared governance found its way into the healthcare and nursing arenas as a form of participative management. It engaged self-managed work teams and grew out of the dissatisfaction nurses were experiencing with the institutions in which they practiced (McDonagh, Rhodes, Sharkey, & Goodroe, 1989; O'May & Buchan, 1999; Porter-O'Grady, 1995).

The professional practice environment of nursing care has shifted dramatically over the past generation (American Association of Colleges of Nurses [AACN], 2002; American Organization of Nurse Executives, 2000; Institutes of Medicine, 2011). Rapid advances are occurring in:

+ Biotechnology and cyberscience

+ Disease prevention, patient safety, and management

+ Relationship-based care

+ Patients' roles in their healthcare (i.e., active partners and not just passive recipients)

Economic constraints related to service reimbursement and corporatism have forced healthcare systems to cost save by:

+ Downsizing the professional workforce

+ Changing staffing mixes

+ Restructuring and/or reorganizing services

+ Reducing support services for patient care

+ Moving patients more rapidly to alternative care settings or discharge

Poor collaboration and ineffective communication among healthcare providers eventuate in sometimes devastating medical errors. The struggle to provide safe, quality care in the highly stressful—and sometimes highly charged—work environment today has resulted in limited success in recruitment and retention of qualified nurses nationwide (AACN, 2002; Kohn, Corrigan, & Donaldson, 1999; Weinberg, 2003).

Shared Governance and Professional Nursing Practice Models

As economic realities shift and change, so does nursing practice. Tim Porter-O'Grady (1987) observed the following: "Reorganization in healthcare institutions is currently the rule rather than the exception. All healthcare participants are attempting to strategically position themselves in the marketplace. What do these changes mean for nursing? How can nursing best respond?" (p. 281). The relevance of developing an effective professional nursing practice model for an economically constrained healthcare system to achieve positive outcomes, build workplace advocacy, and provide needed resources and support to improve recruitment and retention of a shrinking nurse workforce continues to be an even greater challenge today (Barden, 2009; Institutes of Medicine, 2011; Monaghan & Swihart, 2010; Porter-O'Grady & Malloch, 2010a; Swihart, 2006).

Anthony (2004) describes some of the nursing models that have evolved to provide structure and context for care delivery in the reshaping of professional nursing practice:

- Those based on patient care assignment (i.e., team nursing)

- Accountability systems (i.e., primary care nursing)

- Managed care (i.e., case management)

- Shared governance, based on professional autonomy and participatory, or shared, decision-making (i.e., relationship-based care)

Koloroutis (2004) presents the integrated work of nurse leaders, researchers, and authors who have worked with a global community of healthcare organizations over the past 25 years. The result is a nursing model for transforming practice that lends itself effectively to shared governance versus self-governance (see Figure 1.2 for self-governance vs. shared governance) in today's complex healthcare systems: relationship-based care (RBC).

Figure 1.2

SELF-GOVERNANCE VS. SHARED GOVERNANCE

Centralized Interactions

(Self-Governance)

Position-based

Distant from point of care/service

Hierarchical communication

Limited staff input

Separates responsibility/managers
    are accountable

We/they work environment

Divided goals/purpose

Independent activities/tasks

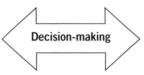

Decision-making

Decentralized Interactions

(Shared Governance)

Knowledge-based

Occurs at point of care/service

Direct communication

High staff input

Integrates equity, accountability, and authority
    for staff and managers

Synergistic work environment

Cohesive goals/purpose, ownership

Collegiality, collaboration, partnership

The RBC model embraces a philosophical foundation and operational framework for providing nursing services through relationships in a caring and healing environment that embodies the concepts of partnership, equity, accountability, and ownership in shared governance.

Shared decision-making occurs best in a decentralized organizational structure where those at the point of service are granted the autonomy and authority to make and determine the appropriateness of their own decisions. "When staff members are clear about their roles, responsibilities, authority, and accountability, they have greater confidence in their own judgments and are more willing to take ownership for decision making at the point of care" (Koloroutis, 2004, p. 72). Decentralized decision-making is most successful when *responsibility*, *authority*, and *accountability* (R+A+A) are clearly delineated and assigned (Wright, 2002) in shared governance.

Responsibility

Responsibility is the clear and specific allocation of duties to achieve desired results. Assignment of responsibility is a two-way process. Responsibility is visibly given and visibly accepted. Acceptance is the essence of responsibility. However, individuals cannot accept responsibility without a level of authority.

Authority

Authority is the right to act and make decisions in the areas where one is given and accepts responsibility. When people are asked to share in the work, they must know their level of authority in which to carry out that work. *Levels of authority* are the right to act in areas one is given and accept authority based on the situation and must be given to those asked to take on responsibility. There are four levels of authority (ways to be clear in communication and delegation of that authority; Wright, 2002):

- Data gathering: "Get information, bring it back to me, and I will decide what to do with it." Example, *Please go down and see if Mr. Jones has a headache and come back and tell me what he says.*

- Data gathering + recommendations: "Get the information (collect the data), look at the situation and make some recommendations, and I will pick from one of those recommendations what we will do next. I still decide." Example, *Please go down and see if Mr. Jones has a headache and come back and tell me what you would recommend that I give him.*

- Data gathering + recommendations [pause] + act: "Get the information (collect the data), look at the situation and make some recommendations, and pick one that you will do. But before you carry it out, I want you to stop (pause) and check with me before you do it." The pause is not necessarily for approval. It is more of a double-check to make sure everything was considered before proceeding. Example, *Please go down and see if Mr. Jones has a headache, come back and tell me what you would recommend for him, and then take care of him for me.*

- Act and inform/update: "Do what needs to be done and tell me what happened or update me later." There is no pause before the action. Example, *Please take care of Mr. Jones for me.*

Accountability

Accountability begins when one reviews and reflects on his or her own actions and decisions, and culminates with a personal assessment that helps determine the best actions to take in the future.

For example, in shared governance, a nurse manager is accountable for patient care delivery in his or her area of responsibility. The manager does not do all the tasks but does provide the resources direct-care nurses need and ensures that patient care delivery is done effectively by all staff members. In that patient care area, the nurse manager is accountable for setting the direction, looking at past decisions, and evaluating outcomes. Bedside nurses are accountable for the overall care outcomes of assigned groups of patients for the time period they are there and for overseeing the big picture; however, other people (dieticians, therapists, pharmacists, laboratory technicians, and other healthcare providers) share in the responsibility for the subsequent tasks in meeting patients' needs.

Although definitions, models, structures, and principles of shared governance (sometimes called *collaborative governance, participatory governance, shared or participatory leadership, staff empowerment,* or *clinical governance*) vary, the outcomes are consistent. The evidence suggests implementation of shared governance and shared decision-making processes result in:

- Increased nurse satisfaction with shared decision-making related to increased responsibility combined with appropriate authority and accountability

- Increased professional autonomy with higher staff and nurse manager retention

- Greater patient and staff satisfaction

- Improved patient care outcomes

- Better financial states due to cost savings and cost reductions

Shared Governance and Relational Partnerships

> The best [leader] is the one who has sense enough to pick good [people] to do what he/she wants done, and self-restraint enough to keep from meddling with them while they do it.
>
> – *Theodore Roosevelt*

Professional nurses long ago identified shared governance as a key indicator of excellence in nursing practice (McDonagh, Rhodes, Sharkey, & Goodroe, 1989; Metcalf & Tate, 1995; Porter-O'Grady, 1987, 2001, 2004, 2009a, 2009b, 2009c). Porter-O'Grady (2001) described shared governance as a management process model for providing a structure for organizing nursing work within organizational settings. It allows strategies for empowering nurses to express and manage their practice with a greater degree of professional autonomy. Personal and professional accountability are respected and supported within the organization. Leadership support for point-of-care nurses enables them to maintain quality nursing practice, job satisfaction, and financial viability when partnership, equity, accountability, and ownership are in place (Anthony, 2004; Green & Jordan, 2002; Koloroutis, 2004; Page, 2004; Porter-O'Grady, 2003a, 2003b; Porter-O'Grady & Malloch, 2010a, 2010b, 2010c).

Today's transformational relationship-based healthcare creates a new paradigm with different goals and objectives in organizational learning environments driven by technology. Leaders, administrators, and employees are learning and implementing new ways of providing care, new technologies, and new ways of thinking and working. In the process, they recognize more and more that the nurse at the point of service is key to organizational success associated with changing the environments of care.

Nurses, managers, interprofessional partners (i.e., physicians, professional nurses, pharmacists), and organizational leaders must be prepared for new roles, new relationships, and new ways of managing. Shared governance is about moving from a traditional hierarchical model to a relational partnership model of nursing practice (see Figure 1.3).

Successful relational partnerships in collaborative interprofessional and interdisciplinary practice require understanding the roles of each partner. If the partners are not aware of what each brings to that relationship, they will have considerable problems collaborating, acting responsibly, and being accountable for decisions and care. Therefore, relational partnerships can be a complex and challenging framework for the shared governance professional nursing practice model (Green & Jordan, 2004; Koloroutis, 2004; Porter-O'Grady, 2002; Porter-O'Grady & Hitchings, 2005; Porter-O'Grady & Malloch, 2010a).

Figure 1.3	FROM HIERARCHY TO RELATIONAL PARTNERSHIP	
From HIERARCHY	to	RELATIONAL PARTNERSHIP
Independence		Interdependence
Hierarchical relationship		Collegial relationship
Parallel functioning		Team functioning
Medical plan		Patient's plan
Resisting change		Leading change
Competing		Partnering
Indirect communication		Direct communication

The key provider at point of service, the direct-care nurse, moves from the bottom to the center of the organization, becoming the only one who matters in a service-based organization, the one providing the care. Nurses are the frontline employees who do the work and connect the organization to the recipient of its service at the point of care. An entirely different sense and set of variables now affect the design of the organization. The paradigm at point of care has shifted to a relationship-based, staff-centered, patient-focused professional nursing practice model of care in which nurse managers or supervisors assume the role of servant leaders managing resources and outcomes within the context of relational partnerships (Nightingale, 1992).

Patient-centered care differs from patient-focused care. The Institute for Healthcare Improvement (IHI) describes patient-centered care in the following way:

Care that is truly patient-centered considers patients' cultural traditions, their personal preferences and values, their family situations, and their lifestyles. It makes the patient and their loved ones an integral part of the care team who collaborate with healthcare professionals in making clinical decisions. Patient-centered care puts responsibility for important aspects of self-care and monitoring in patients' hands—along with the tools and support they need to carry out that responsibility. Patient-centered care ensures that transitions between providers, departments, and healthcare settings are respectful, coordinated, and efficient. When care is patient centered, unneeded and unwanted services can be reduced. (IHI, 2011)

IHI supports shared governance in recognizing the multifaceted challenge in advancing patient-centered care, encouraging organizations to identify best practices and systems changes in three areas:

1.   Involve patients and families in the design of care

2.   Reliably meet patient's needs and preferences

3.   Participation in informed shared decision-making

Healthcare research is guiding the development of initiatives for "reorganizing the delivery of healthcare services around what makes the most sense for patients" (Institute for Medicine, 2001, 2011, p. 51). A few examples of patient-centered care initiatives include:

+   Patient-centered medical homes

+   Transforming care at the bedside

+   Primary care (rather than specialty physician care)

+ Nurse midwives and birth centers

+ Parish nursing

+ Telehealth

+ Community outreach (e.g., Program for All-Inclusive Care for Elders; *www.npaonline.org*)

+ The transitional care model (Institute of Medicine, 2011)

Patient-focused care refers to the caregiver's ability to focus his or her education, experience, and expertise on caring for the patient at the point of service and facilitate organizational and community patient-centered care. To do this, caregivers must have managers who are servant leaders, functioning differently in newly delineated roles (as agent or representative, advocate, ambassador, executor, intermediary, negotiator, proctor, promoter, steward, deputy, and emissary) and transforming practice settings in which patient-focused care occurs. Relational partnerships are built with equity, wherein the value of each of the participants is based on contributions to the relationship rather than on positions within the healthcare system.

Although direct-care nurses and staff are key to *recruiting* other nurses, managers are key to *retaining* them. Collateral and equity-based process models of shared governance define employees by the work they support in regard to each other rather than by their location or position in the system. For example, the manager in the servant, or transformational, leader role provides human and material resources, support, encouragement, and boundaries for the direct-care nurse in the service-provider role. Direct-care nurses, then, are accountable for key roles, decisions, and critical patient care outcomes around practice, quality, and competency. Strong interprofessional collaborations with diverse professional perspectives based on variances in education, experience, and philosophy are essential to be successful in providing point of care services. For example,

+ RNs bring a holistic (whole-istic) approach to care, managing diseases and disorders while considering psychosocial, spiritual, family, and community perspectives

+ Pharmacists bring expertise in pharmacodynamics

+ Physicians bring a more focused approach to diagnostically managing diseases and disorders with expertise in physiology, disease pathways, and treatments (Institute of Medicine, 2011)

Shared governance as an organizational management process model for reshaping nursing practice and decision-making requires a transformational shift with strategic change in organizational culture and leadership through collaboration with interprofessional partners and interdisciplinary team members. Implementation demands a significant realignment in how leaders, employees, and systems transition into new relationships, responsibilities, and accountabilities. It begins with operationalizing the definitions and objectives, building relationships, and creating the design.

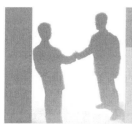

DESIGN A STRUCTURE TO SUPPORT SHARED GOVERNANCE

LEARNING OBJECTIVES

After reading this chapter, the participant should be able to:

- Identify five characteristics that shared governance structures have in common

- Discuss the basic guidelines for forming the governance bodies in shared governance

- Compare and contrast four structural process models of shared governance

The loftier the building, the deeper must the foundation be laid.

– *Thomas Kempis*

Direct-care nurses work closely with an ever-widening network of internal and external stakeholders, healthcare providers, and systems to meet the challenges of today's practice settings and provide safe, effective, quality care. They pull information from multiple sources to facilitate the interrelationships and collaborations among professionals and settings, and for care delivery within the larger organization and communities of practice. For example, when moving patients from the unit (microsystem) through the organization and into the community (macrosystems), direct-care nurses might collaborate with several departments for related services (e.g., pharmacy and social services, mesosystems) prior to discharge, especially if the patient is homeless (see Figures 2.1 and 2.2).

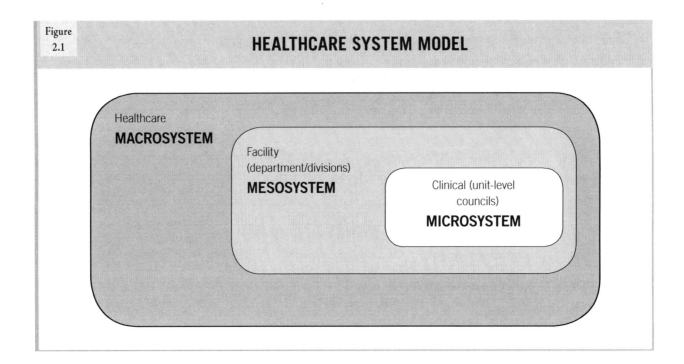

Figure
2.1

HEALTHCARE SYSTEM MODEL

Healthcare
MACROSYSTEM

Facility
(department/divisions)
MESOSYSTEM

Clinical (unit-level
councils)
MICROSYSTEM

Every model, structure, or process of shared governance looks different when appropriately implemented at each of these levels of the organization. The unique character of the organization, its mission, and its staff will yield a foundational organization management process model reflective of the depth and importance of nursing practice and leadership contributions in that organization.

However, there are many features of shared governance that are similar enough to provide some guidance in designing a structure to support shared governance in nursing (Porter-O'Grady, 2004). (See expanded bibliography for many other excellent resources for designing and implementing a shared governance organization management process model.)

All shared governance structures have the following characteristics in common:

+ There is no one way to design or structure a shared governance management process model.

+ Shared governance is grounded in clinical practice at the unit (microsystem) level.

+ Nursing staff are responsible, accountable, and have authority over all decisions related to professional nursing practice (practice, quality, and competence).

 SHARED GOVERNANCE, SECOND EDITION

Figure 2.2	SYSTEM DESCRIPTION	

Organizational level	Description	Teams
Healthcare macrosystem	Whole organization; communities of practice; teams focus on systems, strategic planning, resources allocations (human, material, and fiscal), professional governance, and relationships within the whole organization and communities of practice at local, national, and global levels	Nursing services; senior leaders: CEO, chief operations officer, chief financial officer, chief marketing officer, chief nursing officer, chief information officer; internal and external stakeholders
Facility (departments/ divisions) mesosystem	Major divisions/systems; teams focus on systems and relationships, the structure, framework, and context that support the team's activities (e.g., shared governance, risk management, quality systems, human resources, fiscal services); teams build and sustain professional relationships, interactions, and connections among team members, other teams, and the services they provide to achieve clinical and service-related outcomes	Nursing, medicine, pharmacy, social services, dietetics, laboratory services, environmental management services, radiology, physical and occupational health, rehabilitation, surgery, critical care, informatics, women's health, nursery, pediatrics, and other clinical and departmental service lines
Clinical (unit-level council) microsystem	Frontline nursing units; smaller functional units and teams who focus on specific functions and activities that are the work of the organization at the point of service or care; work collaboratively to facilitate, improve, and advance relationships and services provided by the interdisciplinary team members and interprofessional partners	Nurses, nurse managers, social services/ social workers, pharmacists, physicians, clinical nurse leaders, case managers, clinical nurse specialists, educators and staff development specialists, chaplains and clinical spiritual leaders/pastors, risk managers, and others, including patients and families

Adapted from Monaghan, H. M., & Swihart, D. L. (2010). Clinical Nurse Leader: Transforming Practice, Transforming Care. A Model for the Clinician at the Point of Care. *Sarasota, FL: Visioning Healthcare, Inc.*

- Direct-care nurses are elected to the positions they hold in the shared governance structure by their peers rather than appointed by management.

- Management cannot remove an elected staff representative except as an official action against the employee (e.g., substandard work performance, unethical conduct, failure to perform assigned duties related to job description).

- Shared governance needs to be implemented servicewide at the mesosystem level rather than unit by unit at the microsystem level, thereby creating silos.

- Unit-level operational processes are defined in the unit by the direct-care nurses.

- Direct-care nurses drive the structuring of the shared governance process.

- Management, in the servant leader role, provides the support, encouragement, resources (financial, human, and material), training, and boundaries (organizational and management) necessary for success.

- A coordinating group composed of staff and management provides guidance about issues affecting the department of nursing, communicating the organization's strategic plan, developing shared governance bylaws, approving departmental expenditures or budgets, and/or helping determine accountabilities for appropriate groups and/or members within the shared governance structure.

- It is responsibility- and accountability-based, defined by what nurses do, how they do it, and the outcomes expected from nursing practice at point of care.

- Shared governance is bylaws- or rules-driven. Some units will use project charters (or charters) instead of bylaws. In current usage among many healthcare organizations, a charter is essentially a description of the scope, purpose and/or objectives, and participation guidelines for a committee or council. It identifies and provides a preliminary delineation of roles and responsibilities of participants and stakeholders, defines the authority and duties of the leadership, and serves as a reference of authority for the committee or council. Though similar to bylaws in many ways, a charter is usually considered a more flexible, less formal set of rules, with voting often by consensus, and rarely incorporates parliamentary procedure.

    SHARED GOVERNANCE, SECOND EDITION

Effective shared governance:

* Transforms the organization to a practice model of shared decision-making in a decentralized relational partnership with individual professional responsibility, accountability, and authority over practice decisions at point of service

* Empowers the staff in unexpected ways, such as nontraditional involvement in operations and decision-making

* Shifts some of the accountability historically or traditionally part of the management role or owned by the organization to direct-care nurses

* Shared decision-making means many participants undertake multiple essential roles that are mutual in their exercise and on which each partner depends

* When shared governance is implemented effectively, it affects the organization as a whole, division-wide and at unit level

Basic Requirements of All Shared Governance Systems

There are four elements that are essential to the successful implementation of shared governance in the earliest stages of process development:

1. A committed nurse executive must be invested in process empowerment and willing to undertake the efforts and energy necessary to implement shared governance.

2. A strong management team is essential in terms of commitment to one another, to nursing, to the organization, and to building the structure and implementing the process.

3. The process cannot be implemented if employees do not have a basic understanding of shared governance and can build on that understanding with a working knowledge of what is to be accomplished. There must be a clear destination.

4. The plan and timeline for implementation are critical for benchmarking and charting progress points.

Guidelines for forming the governance bodies:

+ A decision-making group is empowered to make decisions that form a baseline for thinking organizationally when implementing shared governance.

+ Create an appropriate size group (usually seven to 10 participants and generally no more than 14 to 15) to facilitate effective group decision-making. It generally requires about seven people to represent the organization or service line (e.g., nursing) equitably. The presence of more than 15 participants reduces the group's ability to reach decisions or consensus and move the agenda and work forward.

+ Decisional groups must be accountability-based.

+ Within the organization, all groups, committees, and task forces relate to governance bodies or councils.

+ Communication within and across all groups, committees, task forces/teams, and governing councils is critical to the success of implementation and ongoing operations of the shared governance management process model.

Structural Process Models of Shared Governance

Four structural models of shared governance have emerged in America in the past 40 years (Anthony, 2004; Green & Jordon, 2004; Porter-O'Grady, 1986, 1987, 1991; Porter-O'Grady & Hitchings, 2005): (1) congressional, (2) councilor, (3) administrative, and (4) unit level. All four models are based on essentially the same principles but reflect differing specific characteristics depending on the intention of the model, the design and structure of the organization, and the services building it.

Congressional model of shared governance

One of the first models developed, the congressional model of shared governance reflects primarily a specific nursing orientation to its design. This model features a staff congress comprised of an elected president and a cabinet or senate of officers as well as all the professional staff, including management and direct-care nurses, who oversee the operations of a unit, area, or department. The various committees of the congress, who are delegated by the congress to make certain decisions and to have certain powers, are selected out of that congress and report back to the cabinet or senate. The congress defines its accountabilities and assigns those accountabilities to various committees of the congress. See Figure 2.3 for a diagram of the congressional model (adapted from Porter-O'Grady, 1991).

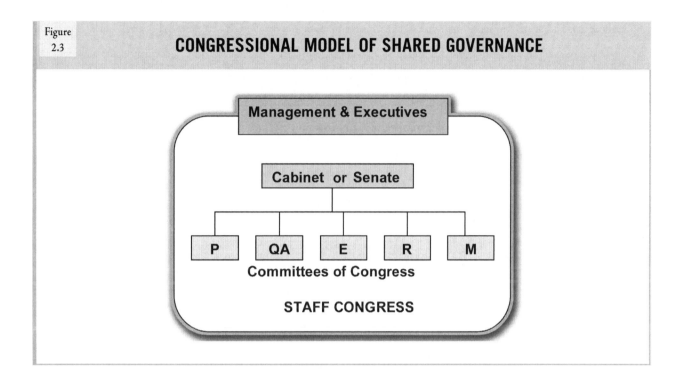

Figure 2.3

CONGRESSIONAL MODEL OF SHARED GOVERNANCE

Management & Executives

Cabinet or Senate

P | QA | E | R | M

Committees of Congress

STAFF CONGRESS

Five basic accountabilities emerge from the committees of congress:

1. Practice

2. Quality assurance/improvement

3. Professional development/education

4. Research

5. Management

These accountabilities reflect the basic professional accountabilities of the disciplines. The work of the nursing organization is carried out in the committees of congress and disseminated to direct-care nurses and other stakeholders from there.

Councilor model of shared governance

The councilor model is very similar to the congressional model and is one of the most commonly used models in healthcare. It consists of councils on clinical practice, quality assurance, management, research, advocacy, and staff development/education. The term *council* is used to differentiate the work of the shared governance organizational management process teams from the committees and task groups, which are usually groups of people chosen or appointed to perform a specified service or function. For example, all unit-level decisions related to professional nursing practice, quality, and competence are given over to a unit council. However, inquiries and decisions relative to policies and procedures are given over to the standards of care committee.

The councils are empowered by the nursing staff to perform the basic accountabilities identified in the congressional model: practice, quality assurance/improvement, research, staff development/education, and management. However, the structure is slightly different. Councils are empowered with the authority rather than the congress. Each council is delegated by the organization with accountability and authority for decisions that fall within the context of that council. For example, all practice decisions belong to the practice council, all quality assurance/improvement decisions belong to the quality council, all professional development and education belong to the professional development council, and so on.

With the exception of the management council and the research council, all councils are made up predominantly of direct-care nurses. Direct-care nurses make up about 90% of the councils and make the decisions related to accountabilities for practice, quality, and competency that are staff-based. In that way, actual accountability shifts from the traditional management framework to a staff framework as determined by the locus of control or the legitimate place of that accountability. For example, practice should always be in the hands of the practitioners; therefore, practice decisions are undertaken by practicing clinicians who are at the point of service or care. Responsibility, authority, and accountability for those decisions, policies, and outcomes rest with them. See Figure 2.4 for a diagram of the councilor model (adapted from Porter-O'Grady, 1991).

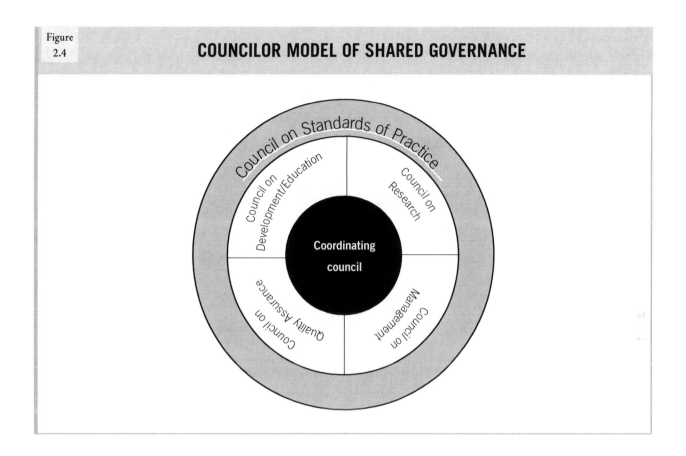

Figure 2.4

COUNCILOR MODEL OF SHARED GOVERNANCE

Administrative model of shared governance

The administrative model follows more traditional organizational lines of management and practice with each having separate groups that address specific functions and accountabilities. The model resembles a more traditional hierarchy with two structural units, management and clinical, which are generally aligned in a top-down relationship, although the members in both tracks may include both managers and staff as implementation advances. All work is done by committees and reported back to the overarching council or committee. The executive committee may make decisions on information provided for all clinical issues that concern more than one committee along either or both tracks. See Figure 2.5 for a diagram of the administrative model (adapted from Hess [2009] and Porter-O'Grady [1991]).

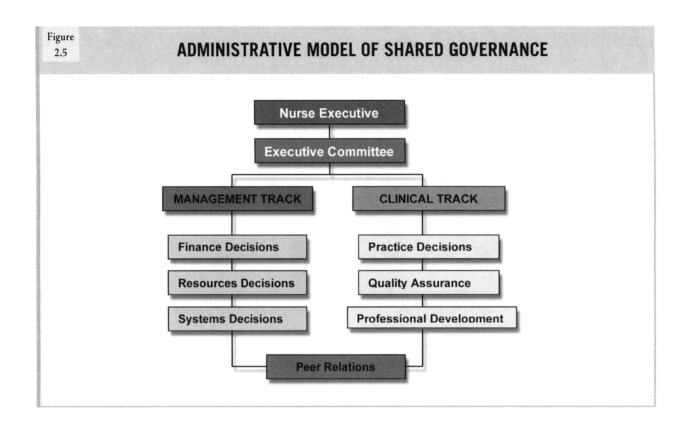

Figure 2.5

ADMINISTRATIVE MODEL OF SHARED GOVERNANCE

The structural familiarity in communicating decisions upward is a key characteristic of this model. The decision-making groups are composed of at least 50% staff or a representative proportion of staff to management depending on the degree of organizational commitment to direct-care nurse participation in shared governance.

Unit-level model of shared governance

The unit-level model is rarely used. (Note: This is a structural model and is not to be confused with the unit-level councils in the councilor model.) The design principles are similar but the structure is fundamentally different. The culture of the unit gives it form. Members define their own basic accountabilities; units become entities unto themselves and make decisions about what they do and how they do it that may not impact the organization outside of the unit.

One of the problems with this model might be individual, insular, cultural application of shared governance with no integrating or coordinating principles from the division as a whole giving it guidance. Individual units may build powerful decision-making models that direct-care nurses exemplify and appreciate but may operate to jeopardize the structures of the whole division, service, or organization.

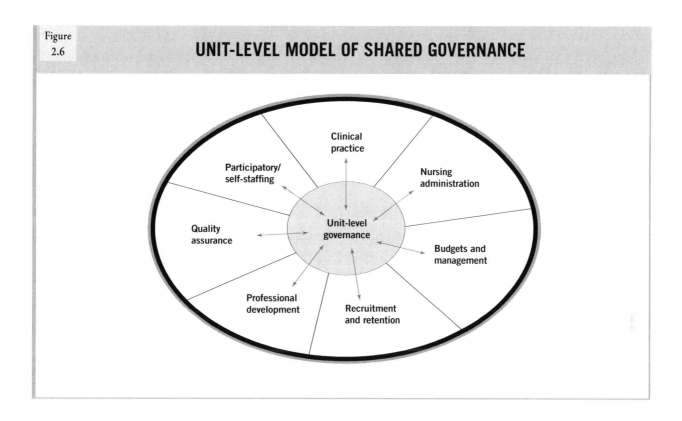

Figure
2.6

UNIT-LEVEL MODEL OF SHARED GOVERNANCE

However, the accountabilities defined in this model do work well when adapted to the councilor model for unit-level councils working in tandem, or in partnership, with the meso- and macrosystems of the organization (see Appendix 3, unit council worksheet). See Figure 2.6 for a diagram of a unit-level model of shared governance (adapted from Hess [2009] and Porter-O'Grady [1991]).

Shared governance demands an investment of effort and time by all partners from all levels of the healthcare system. As nurses reshape the professional practice community, the necessity for a relational partnership between management and direct-care nurses in decision-making affects the design and structuring of care in the professional practice environment. In the process, knowledge of the basic concepts and a commitment to them is a prerequisite to the design and implementation processes.

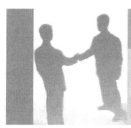

BUILD A STRUCTURE TO SUPPORT SHARED GOVERNANCE

After reading this chapter, the participant should be able to:

- Identify four strategic changes related to implementation of shared governance

- Describe the roles and responsibilities of a design team for implementation of shared governance

- Discuss the purpose of bylaws and articles and how they are established when formalizing the shared governance structure

Implementing Shared Governance

> The greatest amount of wasted time is the time not getting started.
>
> – *Dawson Trotman*

Venner Farley (2000) observed, "For nurses, re-structuring means change ... Nurses must have a great capacity for change in order to accept the challenges of creating our future. The rewards will be substantial: autonomy and independence within a framework of collaboration and colleagueship" (pp. 24–25). She encouraged nurses to begin thinking and behaving differently as they embrace change along five parameters (p. 24):

- Face reality as it is

- Be open and honest with everyone

- Don't manage ... lead

- Change before you have to

- Recognize that nursing and nurses must seek and maintain a competitive advantage

Leading Strategic Change

> One of the reasons people don't achieve their dreams is that they desire to
> change their results without changing their thinking.
>
> – *John C. Maxwell*

The changes in pace, demand, technological complexity, and patient populations today are greater than ever before. Consequently, the costs of resistance to those changes and failure to implement collaborative partnerships in shared decision-making can be catastrophic. Nurses have choices about where and how they will work. They are no longer willing to work for authoritarian top-down management systems. They are choosing ANCC Magnet Recognition Program® (MRP) hospitals with high-involvement shared governance structures and processes and evolving professional nursing practice models. Strategic changes related to implementation of shared governance include structural changes, organizational changes, cultural changes, and individual changes, such as those listed in Figure 3.1 (Porter-O'Grady, 2004).

Figure 3.1		

FOUR TYPES OF STRATEGIC CHANGES RELATED TO IMPLEMENTING SHARED GOVERNANCE

Structural changes	Individual changes
Multidisciplinary work flow patterns	New realities
Communication structures	Degrees of change
Ongoing assessment of work patterns	Sound practice standards
Access to resources	Clear and strong ethics
Investment at all levels of the organization	Dialogue and communication
Increasing dependence on interdependence	Honesty and integrity
Role definitions and descriptions	Curiosity and creativity
Movement away from status determinations	Willingness to seek/abide by consensus
Based on accountabilities, not hierarchies	Able to express concerns and ideas
	Structured risk-taking
	Competency
	Varying degrees of involvement
	Increasing self-confidence
Organizational changes	**Cultural changes**
Salaried work roles	Reward systems altered
Reward systems; achievement rewards	Continuous management development
Gainsharing strategies	Continuous leadership (manager and staff) development
Role accountabilities clarification	Career enhancement programs
Partnerships	Hiring and termination processes
Mentoring and precepting roles	Staff role ownership, including position descriptions
Variable loci of leadership roles	Benefits programs
Work design (nurse driven)	Unit/service programs vs. divisional ones
Patient-centered care redesign	
New orientation and socialization processes	

A fundamental part of undertaking the processes associated with implementing shared governance and achieving successful outcomes is grounded in leading strategic change (Black & Gregersen, 2008), which becomes the driving force for defining and restructuring professional relationships. Every decision and action is set on some idea or theory that events or actions will result in predetermined outcomes. These are mental maps—beliefs about cause and effect—that guide people's decisions and behaviors. Most mental maps were forged in experience.

When people work successfully together in particular ways to make recurring decisions and complete repetitive tasks, they begin to assume that these are the ways things should be done. This works well *except* when things change. Black and Gregersen (2008) offer insights for changing mind maps that prevent people from changing and/or from maintaining the changes in place, one of the greatest obstacles to implementing shared governance in professional practice settings. Change the individual, and the organization will follow. Change is not easy. It begins and ends with the mental maps about the organization and the jobs employees entertain in their heads. If those maps cannot be rewritten, if the brain barrier cannot be broken, there is nothing new for hearts and hands to follow. Without a compelling case for change, staff-centered, patient-focused, relationship-based care in shared decision-making will not follow.

Resistance to change is fundamental and biologically hard-wired into humans. We are programmed for survival, to resist random change, and to maintain stability and sameness. Black and Gregersen (2008) call this the "map-hugging dynamic" (p. 3). Nurses encountering shared governance for the first time may have difficulty letting go of old maps and ways of doing things.

The fundamental change process or cycle is based on the 80/20 principle, which says that 80% of the work comes from 20% of the workers. This explains why so many change initiatives fail: only 20% of the employees capture 80% of the picture of strategic change. Black and Gregersen (2003, p. 13) identify four stages of successful strategic change:

  + Stage 1: Do the right thing and do it well

  + Stage 2: Discover that the right thing is now the wrong thing

  + Stage 3: Do the new right thing, but do it poorly at first

  + Stage 4: Eventually do the new right thing well

Leading strategic change in transforming professional nursing practice through shared governance and the essentials of the principles identified in the ANCC Magnet Recognition Program® requires organizations to channel efforts in training, educating, and empowering others to get ahead of the change curve to master anticipatory change rather than subject themselves constantly to reactionary or crisis change (McClure & Hinshaw, 2002).

So how exactly does remapping change work? Black and Gregersen (2008) discuss three primary brain barriers leading to failed change and the keys to successfully overcoming those barriers and delivering strategic change in healthy organizations.

1. **Brain barrier: failure to see the need for change when what they have already been doing seems to still be working for them**

    +   **Contrast.** Look at key contrasts at how strategies, structures, cultural values, processes, technologies, practice models, and approaches to nursing leadership that worked in the past are no longer effective in the present or appropriate for the future.

    +   **Confrontation.** Leaders may have to confront nurses with clear and compelling evidences between past, present, and future contrasts to help them see before they can move to change. They cannot—they will not—change if they do not see the need to do so.

2. **Brain barrier: failure to move after they see the need to change because they do not believe in the new path, their ability to walk it, or the rewarding outcomes of the journey and destination**

    +   **Destinations.** Make sure everyone sees the destination clearly to gain belief in the move to shared governance. People cannot change if they do not see the destination clearly or understand where they are going.

    +   **Resources.** Give them the skills, resources, and tools they need to reach the destination and participate in shared governance.

    +   **Rewards.** Deliver valuable rewards along the journey that have meaning to the employee. People value many things. The ARCTIC assessment tool (see Figure 3.2) can help identify rewards that would have greater meaning to people and more power to move change and successfully implement shared governance (adapted from Black & Gregersen [2008, p. 84]).

<table>
<tr><td colspan="2" align="center">Figure 3.2</td></tr>
</table>

ARCTIC ASSESSMENT TOOL

ARCTIC	Rewards
Achievement	• Accomplishment: the need to meet or beat goals, to do better in the future than one has done in the past • Competition: the need to compare one's performance with that of others and do better than others do
Relations	• Approval: the need to be appreciated and recognized by others • Belonging: the need to feel a part of and accepted by the group
Conceptual Thinking	• Problem solving: the need to confront problems and create answers • Coordination: the need to relate pieces and integrate them into a whole
Improvement	• Growth: the need to feel continued improvement and growth as a person, not just improved results • Exploration: the need to move into unknown territory for discovery
Control	• Competence: the need to feel personally capable and competent • Influence: the need to influence others' opinions and actions

3. **Brain barrier: failure to finish because they are tired and lost**

   • **Champions.** Trained and motivated change champions are needed close to the action in every practice setting from the moment that the decision to change is implemented.

   • **Charting.** Progress must be measured at all levels in the organization and reported. Performance—good, bad, or indifferent—needs to be communicated to staff members. Successful change requires monitoring and communicating at the individual level.

Leading strategic change by breaking the three brain barriers involves remapping old behaviors and guiding staff through the process individually first to ultimately impact the organization as a whole. Failure to see is a problem of entrenched, successful maps; high contrast and confrontation is needed to break through this barrier. Failure to move happens when smart people resist going from doing the wrong thing well to doing the right new thing poorly. It takes ensuring the destination is clear, resources are in place, and valued rewards are provided to break through this barrier. Finally, failure to finish is a consequence of nurses getting tired and lost. Therefore, they do not go fast enough or far enough. Champions and open communication about progress, good or bad, is critical for breaking through this barrier.

Change is constant. It is the only real absolute in healthcare. Shared governance cannot be successful until all partners come together on how to lead strategic change. Once the barriers to leading strategic change are understood, Dr. Michael Peterman (2011), an organizational development psychologist and change management architect for the Veterans Health Administration Office of Clinical Consultation and Compliance, recommends using a change management team to:

- Develop a vision and strategy for change

- Design and manage the change process

- Guide execution of the strategy

- Make the case for change

- Build motivation to change

- Enable and support change

- Anticipate and address sources of resistance (What are the organizational and individual forces opposing and supporting change leading to successful implementation of shared governance?)

- Reinforce and anchor change

- Provide accurate and timely communication

Making the case for change

Why should I change? *Why* before how …

Make a compelling case, the most important part of any major change, and teach representatives from each unit council how to present it. Peterman (2011) describes components for building a compelling case for change:

- Ask if change is dependent on having a viable solution to the questions

- Describe why the change is a viable solution to the problem at hand

- Describe the nature of the change (i.e., the vision)

- Explain why the change is necessary

- Identify the benefits of change

- Anticipate and address sources of resistance

- Make presentations specific to target audience

- Incorporate feedback from key stakeholders

- Use a credible presenter to deliver the case for change

- Connect shared governance to what people value

- Include feedback from internal and external stakeholders at all levels

- Make sure the message has emotional appeal

- Use tools like metaphors, storytelling and exemplars, and case studies

- Include supporting data

- Communicate the case for change effectively and repeatedly

In the absence of a compelling case for change, motivation will likely be insufficient. Once the case for change has been made and accepted, it is time to move forward with the design, establishment, and maturing of shared governance structures and processes.

Shared Governance Systems: Perspective and Format

Structure the shared governance format and vision carefully. Identify organizational and nursing's purposes, objectives, goals, direction, and strategic plans; reflect the organization's mission; and determine the roles nurses and nurse leaders will have in shared governance: conceptual base, philosophy, objectives, care standards, performance measures, quality assurance/performance improvement, professional development, and practice.

Designing the shared governance process

Select members from nursing service and interdisciplinary teams to form a shared governance design team (or forum, group, steering committee, or coordinating group). They will obtain feedback from leadership and staff; consider nursing's objectives and the organization's goals, mission, and philosophy; and draft a process model for shared governance. The final design will be selected by nursing staff and nursing leadership to represent an integrated process and structure for shared decision-making toward positive patient outcomes. Design the structure and process to address each part of professional nursing practice: quality, competence, and practice.

Although there are four basic structures for shared governance described in the literature, the councilor model (illustrated in Figure 3.3) is currently the most popular model used in nursing practice at point of service (Hess, 2009; Anthony, 2004; Porter-O'Grady, 1991, 2004). Therefore, it will be presented here in greater detail for the purposes of developing the concepts and principles of shared governance implementation more fully.

Implementing a councilor model for shared decision-making

Here are the steps to take for implementing a councilor model:

+ Design a framework for discussing implementation of shared governance and setting the direction for reshaping professional nursing practice.

+ Evaluate the basic structure of the selected model (in this case, the councilor model).

+ Identify and simplify accountability of disciplines. There are five basic constructs that can be separated or combined in the design structure of the governing councils or bodies. All professional committees, task forces, and practice groups will eventually be folded into one or more of these disciplines and become part of a designated governing council.

+ Create a professional overlay for designing individual elements of the structure. The accountabilities (practice, management, quality, education, and research) will be the basis of the formation of the governing councils, whether in five councils or some other designated grouping.

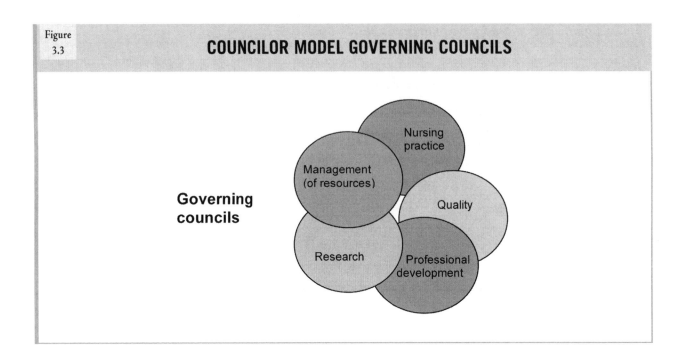

Figure 3.3

COUNCILOR MODEL GOVERNING COUNCILS

Establish a design team

Here are some guidelines for establishing a design team, which can also be known as a steering group or coordinating group:

- **Design team size (limit size to about seven to 15 members):** The larger the group, the less constructive they may be in finding consensus for making and implementing decisions.

- **Design team membership:** The design team mix needs to represent the percentage distribution of the organization of management and direct-care nurses (majority). Drawing from services rather than work units generally establishes a broader group but keeps the team small enough to be effective. Select nurse leaders, direct-care nurses, and interdisciplinary team members so they form a partnership in designing, implementing, and communicating the process elements of shared governance from the beginning.

- **Design team purpose:** Focus on designing the shared governance process structure that will evolve after implementation:

    - The entire design process falls under this group

    - This team coordinates all of the shared governance activities initially

* **Design team goals:** The team is empowered to do the work:

  - Plan shared governance: Define and describe what shared governance is and what it will look like in this organization at the point of service for nurses and nursing leaders. Identify the roles of the interdisciplinary team members, executive leadership, and internal and external stakeholders.

  - Guide implementation: Once the structure is designed and shared governance has been defined in terms of an implementation plan, the design team continues to guide the process. Over time, the design team may change names (e.g., coordinating council, nursing town hall, or nursing forum) and expand functions to facilitate the ongoing progress of shared governance in nursing.

  - Help nursing staff and leaders with transition: Create a timetable for transition. Assess readiness. Complete predetermined activities and provide subsequent activities for group members once councils are established. Develop a mechanism for personal and professional transitioning, a way of acknowledging accomplishments, and a social or symbolic activity for the transition (Porter-O'Grady, 2004).

  - Evaluate progress: Evaluate progress initially, at six months, then annually once shared governance is implemented: where you are, how far you have come, and what has to be done in light of the design or plan you set in motion. This is critical to measuring success (Hess, 1998a, 1998b).

Roles and responsibilities of the design team

* **Learn about shared governance and how it works:** If they are responsible for designing the format for shared governance, they need as much knowledge as possible from the beginning stages through mature development and standardization of practice. Build an information base to understand and structure the work.

* **Select a shared governance process structure or model:** Determine which shared governance structure or model applies to the organization based on its culture, goals, and strategic plan. The structure selected must be a good fit for the organization and for professional nursing practice. Expect this structure to be adapted initially and multiple times as it matures and conforms to the needs of the nurses and the organization with more and more voices represented over time.

+ **Identify tasks and create a timeline:** Focus on what will occur at what time to evaluate elements of the process and ensure that everyone succeeds in finishing assigned tasks. Developing this process is a long-term event. It usually takes three to five years to fully implement an effective, efficiently operating shared governance process model. Each stage of the process builds on previous stages. Evaluating each stage will be preliminary to beginning the next stage. The timeline becomes a guide to successfully implementing the process and to determining where you are along the way. It helps keep the destination visible so that all participants can move to accept and manage the many changes needed for shared governance (Black & Gregersen, 2008; Porter-O'Grady, 1991).

+ **Evaluate goals and process outcomes:** Emphasize goals and anticipated outcomes at the beginning of the process (e.g., higher levels of nurse satisfaction, higher retention rates, increased patient safety outcomes). Measure and evaluate goals intermittently along the way. Design or select tools for measuring progress in shared governance that allow for evaluation and adjustment in the process along the way as outcomes are achieved (see Appendices 1 and 2 for the Index of Professional Governance and Index of Professional Nursing Governance).

Designing governance councils

When establishing the selected shared governance process structure, identify how many councils (bodies or groups) will be created to include all five accountabilities or disciplines. Once the disciplines are accounted for, there is no right or wrong way to design the structure or process. One organization elected to create five governing councils: (1) nursing town hall (management/coordinating council), (2) practice council, (3) quality and research council, (4) professional development council, and (5) unit-level councils, which were connected to each of the other four councils. This allowed nursing to slightly reduce the number of council meetings direct-care nurses would need to attend while still maintaining representation in each governing body. (In this book, a council is described separately for each accountability or discipline for discussion.)

Begin by identifying the outcomes desired. Some organizations establish one council at a time to help employees transition more easily and successfully through the change process. Others establish the governing councils and unit councils together to promote interactivity, communication, and work flow. This book will address the councils and structures one at a time to better describe them in more detail and recommend an order of establishment for those organizations who choose that approach.

1. **Start with the management (coordinating or leadership) council.** Purpose and responsibilities are to provide guidance and linkage to the governing councils and serve as a mechanism for the nurse executive, nurse leaders, and nurse managers to participate in activities related to the provision of nursing care at point of service. The management council deals almost exclusively with resource issues and allocations. The role for nurse leaders and managers in shared governance is primarily servant-based, providing resources, support, opportunities, boundaries, and protection (i.e., from losing needed resources during annual budget allocations) for nursing staff at point of care, thereby freeing staff to focus all of their experience, expertise, and education on caring for the patient and improving patient care outcomes. The manager:

   + Appropriates necessary resources for the professionals in practice (human, fiscal, material, support, and systems)

   + Centers service around the practicing professional at point of care

   + Integrates (links) the shared governance process with the other services and roles

   + Channels information to and from direct-care nurses through unit-level councils to and from nursing and organizational leadership, when appropriate

   + Identifies systems problems and generates necessary responses

   + Communicates encouragement, support, and boundaries (e.g., tells direct-care nurses when there is no budget for new equipment requested by the unit-level council then helps them explore other options for getting the necessary resources)

Management frequently has the greatest amount of growth and change to undergo for shared governance to be successful. Empowered staff members assume new roles of responsibility, authority, equity, accountability, and ownership traditionally belonging to managers that can cause territorial, personality, and role conflicts during implementation of shared decisional processes. Nurse leaders will need educational programs to help them adapt to new behaviors, learn new roles, and develop new skills as their current role evolves from management to servant leadership, a much higher and more demanding form of leading. This will be a challenging process for them. Devoting time and resources to their transitional development in the transformation of their leadership roles is critical.

2. **Establish the unit-level councils.** This usually follows or correlates well with the implementation of the management council. Here is where it all comes together. Purpose and responsibilities are to promote autonomy, equity, partnership, and shared accountability and ownership for unit operations by managing point-of-service care; measuring and documenting patient outcomes (nursing quality indicators); providing orientation, mentorships, and/or preceptorships for new employees, new graduates, and students doing clinical rotations; participating in schedule development; sharing charge nurse responsibilities; conflict resolution and problem solving; assessing and meeting educational needs and unit-specific competencies; engaging in evidence-based practice (research, journal clubs); monitoring unit-specific practice and safety issues (policies, quality improvement, patient safety); and managing unit education (in-services, mandatory training, continuing education).

3. **Develop a practice council.** Purpose and responsibilities are to set the criteria for evidence-based practice consistent with established and/or evolving professional standards and regulating agencies. This council keeps the development of the staff in concert with the changes of management/leadership roles. Most of the other councils' work will depend on the foundational work completed and managed by the practice council, which has the control and authority to make decisions affecting policies and practice for the work that they do:

    +   Define, implement, and maintain practice

    +   Selects theory base

    +   Sets practice standards

    +   Sets performance standards

    +   Defines career advancement

4. **Initiate a quality council.** Purpose and responsibilities are to monitor and evaluate performance and outcome measurements based on evidence-based practice using the best scientific knowledge available, to provide a forum for interdisciplinary team collaboration, and to integrate quality initiatives into practice. The work of the quality council depends on the work of the management and practice councils. For example, the practice council's service standards need to be developed before the quality council can identify and develop measurement standards. Performance standards must be done before developing a performance evaluation system (quality council).

Therefore, it is important to establish a deliberate, step-by-step relationship among the councils and a clear basis on which they can depend for their complementary development.

The goal of shared governance is that ownership and investment of all the workers and the outcome of the work ties back into how we define the work and how performance is measured against that definition. If the staff member defines the work, performs on that definition, and achieves work outcomes, they can also evaluate progress or individual performance related to that work. The quality council:

+ Monitors and measures standards of care. Establishing unit-level clinical quality council champions is one approach to interactive collaboration for continuous quality improvement. Appendixes 30, 31, and 32 are tools used by the staff of the surgical ICU at St. Luke's Health System to establish such champions and orient them to their roles within unit-level councils and in partnership with the governing quality council and the quality management systems.

+ Designs the quality and performance improvement system and dashboards or scorecards.

+ Controls the performance evaluation system (a peer-based process in shared governance, not management-based).

+ Sets the goals for patient care monitoring (defines a standard of care, measures it, reaches it, and changes the standard so nurses work at a higher level of function or outcome).

+ Manages the credentialing and privileging program. Every professional nurse has an obligation for the quality and type of work he or she does. Establishing a peer-based process for new nurses when they first enter the organization that continues throughout their employment helps ensure a good fit with the organization and with nursing service.

5. **Initiate a nursing professional development council.** Purpose and responsibilities are to provide orientation; to assess ongoing learning and competency needs; and to define, implement, and maintain standards, continuing education, and in-services that promote professional and personal growth and ongoing competency of professional nurses and their healthcare team members. The professional development council:

+ Ensures professional competency in ongoing learning activities, the basis of performance measurement over the long-term. This council facilitates implementation of competency mechanisms that ensure a continuous mechanism for education and development is present, is staff-based, and clearly represents the work done rather than some preplanned objective that may or may not reflect the unit-specific needs of the nurses at point of service.

- Develops an effective communication network through each of the councils.

- Manages staff orientation programs and preceptorships, which are critical to the success of new employees (graduate nurses, nurse managers, agency/contract nurses), and unit-specific or clinical orientations.

- Plans quarterly and annual staff meetings:

  - Quarterly meetings: Staff and council members get together to deal with issues of concern to the organization as a whole as it impacts nursing service; to report to the staff what activities they have been involved in; to get feedback from the staff about what is occurring; to relate, communicate, and interact; to look at goals and learning objectives for the year; review activities and the progress of those activities over time; and to deal with operational issues.

  - Annual meetings: Staff and council members look at goals and objectives of the organization, discuss and/or report the annual learning needs assessment and education plan, consider problems and issues of the discipline (education and professional development) as a whole, determine how to fit those issues with the goals of the organization, and review organizational problems and issues affecting the discipline. This is an opportunity to give awards for service and to acknowledge the contributions of those who have acted on behalf of the staff during the previous year. It can be an opportunity for formal and informal communication and celebration.

- Facilitates nursing staff members' access to learning-teaching activities by bringing training to the unit level. Balance, personal growth, and professional development are natural outcomes of shared governance activities. Facilitating unit-level education is a major goal of this council. The learning process, content, and activities become more real and meaningful when applied more directly to professional practice at the point of service.

6. **Establish a research and evidence-based practice council (if applicable).** This council follows the development of the previous two councils, quality and professional development. Not all organizations have well-defined research activities. However, one of the clinical accountabilities in shared governance and part of the MRP journey is research. Professional nurses need to be committed to validating old knowledge and discovering new knowledge, which is an integral part of the research process. Research seeks knowledge that will enhance patient care outcomes, offer a new basis for the work to be done at point of service, and help direct-care nurses develop critical thinking skills, evidence-based practices, and abilities to understand and participate in research at the point of care. This council is a way to formalize that process. It is the last council implemented because it is the most dependent on the other councils being in place and is the most resource dependent.

7. **Create an advocacy council (if applicable).** This council is becoming more embedded in the culture of shared governance models and often works in concert with the professional development council. The advocacy council defines and maintains strategies that support all nursing service employees. Members promote professional advancement, advocacy, and recognitions through communication, coordination, and staff advocacy, recruitment and recognition, and celebratory activities around practice, quality, and competency of nurses at all levels. They work most closely with unit-level councils in identifying needs and developing their activities. Some of those activities include establishing and promoting relationships among all types of community organizations through contributions to patient outcomes and the health of the communities they serve, e.g., providing CPR to the community during an annual CPR day. This council also seeks opportunities to acknowledge nurses in various and substantive ways for their accomplishments, enhancing the image of nursing in the organization and in the community, through awards ceremonies, public announcements of certifications and promotions, and special events, i.e., collecting clothes and toiletries for the homeless. Because of the generally fun and celebratory atmosphere of this council, there are nearly always lots of volunteers to serve on it.

Focus on council membership

When recruiting members for the varied shared governance councils, there are a number of factors to consider: representation, contributions, membership mix, size of councils, length of time of participant service, and meeting times.

1. **Representation:** From a service context, these representatives will speak on behalf of those
    services when decisions have to be made.

2. **Contributions:** Contributions are made by each member over time; work may be assigned to
    members to be done in the meeting or taken back to their units/areas and completed there.
    Reports on tasks and progress are given at each council meeting.

3. **Membership mix:** Staff governance councils (practice, quality, professional development) need
    to be comprised of mostly direct-care nurses, about 70% to 90% clinical staff. The other council
    members should be management or support staff. These are direct-care nurse councils. They
    will make staff decisions that affect clinical practice, quality, and competency. Messages of
    empowerment, equity, autonomy, and accountability are delivered in an effective and clear way
    so that shared decision-making emerges in partnership with the staff and management.

4. **Size of councils:** Number of participants depends on the number of units represented. Usually,
    only seven to 15 members are recommended. However, there are organizations with more
    representatives at the table. It is important that all nursing units/areas have someone at the table
    to represent their voices in the discussions and shared decision-making. The larger the groups,
    though, the more difficult it is to get consensus and make decisions. How to overcome this
    potential obstacle would have to be addressed by the design team when developing initial
    guidelines for the council structures and/or at the beginning of work in larger groups by the
    council members.

5. **Length of time of participant service:** It often takes about a year for a participant to learn
    the roles of assigned councils. Therefore, a two-year term seems to be emerging as the standard
    length of service commitment for each governing council member. With a two-year term, consider
    rotating one-half of the members off one year and the other half off the second year. This rotation
    would provide continuity of process with at least one-half of the members having served for one
    year and able to orient and mentor the oncoming council members. For unit-level councils,
    however, a one-year term seems to be the norm at present.

6. **Meeting times and structures:** How organizations elect to structure their council meetings and
    times will be dependent on factors unique to that staff:

- Some councils meet once a month for eight hours (a full day) to accomplish the tasks of the council. This allows members to focus on the business of the council instead of dividing their attention or concern with the patients or tasks they left on the unit for an hour or two.

- Other councils have a monthly "meeting day" when all councils meet, usually for an hour each, at different times to allow staff members to attend their meetings and return to work around the council meetings. Breaks of 15 to 30 minutes between council meetings allow staff members who serve on more than one council to get to the next one without disrupting or interfering with the work of other councils. For example:

    8 a.m. to 9 a.m.: Management or coordinating council

    9:30 a.m. to 10:30 a.m.: Quality council

    11 a.m. to 12 p.m.: Professional development council

    12:30 p.m. to 1:30 p.m.: Practice council

    2 p.m. to 3 p.m.: Research and evidence-based practice council (if one has been established)

    3:30 p.m. to 4:30 p.m.: Advancements, advocacy, and recognitions council (if one has been established)

- Council meetings *cannot* be optional. Attendance has to be mandatory if direct-care nurses and nursing leadership are to have a voice in shared decision-making and be able to complete and communicate council activities. It is critical that nursing leadership support and facilitate staff attendance at assigned council meetings. It is also important to provide time and opportunity for communication of information and/or data gathering to complete council assignments (e.g., unit-level in-services). These are details to be discussed and resolved by each nurse leader/manager and his or her staff.

Each council is structured with certain accountabilities or disciplines. Staff councils must have the authorities identified that belong to the staff and operate within the staff framework.

Focus on shared governance empowerment process

Each governing council selects a chair from among the membership to provide leadership for the council. For the staff councils, that chair will be selected from among the staff, the research council chair may be management or staff, and the management council selects its own chair. These chairs must be empowered to do the work of managing or leading the councils with the responsibility, authority, equity, ownership, and accountability to make decisions and to act on those decisions. Empowering the chair means the chair of each council will be given certain basic powers secured by the role. It is recommended that the chair will:

1. Be elected by peers

2. Control the agenda

3. Act for the group, speak for the group members, and make decisions for them when the group is not in session

4. Assign group tasks/functions

5. Move the group to decision-making, when discussion indicates a need

6. Accept no additional assignments; this role is extensive enough without additional assignments

7. Remove nonperforming members from the group if necessary

Bylaws and Articles: Formalizing the Shared Governance Structure

> You've got to think about "big things" while you're doing small things,
> so that all the small things go in the right direction.
>
> *– Alvin Toffler*

During the formalization of the shared governance structures, the roles of management and implementation of shared decision-making are established in the clinical and work units of the organization. Principles that underpin shared governance are defined and their application to the organization as a whole are described. Activities after the beginning phases of implementation are completed. This process usually takes from two to three years to be fully established. At the end of that time, identify the activities that provide structure and context to the newly designed professional nursing practice in ways that can be understood and replicated by participants in other parts of the organization.

Bylaws for shared governance process models

Developing and implementing bylaws are generally part of the formalization of the shared governance process (Porter-O'Grady, 1991, 2004). Bylaws may be either descriptive or prescriptive:

+ Prescriptive bylaws set the rules on which an organization will evolve.

+ Descriptive bylaws describe the organization already in place. Many groups prefer descriptive bylaws.

Organizational structure is established based on the design and implementation plan with each part of the structure in place. The bylaws, then, simply define the structure once the implementation process begins. When it occurs and is far enough along to give evidence of the operating structure that the participants want, look specifically at bylaws. (See Appendixes 4, 5, and 6 for samples of bylaws for unit-level councils, with guidelines for shared governance process models, and a structure for the ANCC Magnet Recognition Program®.)

When all the pieces come together, it is important to recognize that the work of the design team (steering council) ends at some point in the implementation process. By the end of the second or third year, the formative design stages of the organization end. It is important to transition to a more legitimate council format to integrate the organizational system before this occurs. The executive council generally emerges from this context.

Emerging executive (or nursing town hall/management or coordinating) council

1. **Move from design team or steering committee to executive/management/coordinating council:** Chairs of the individual councils are elected and nominated to assume leadership roles. Each of these elected chairs becomes a member of the executive council with the chief nurse executive or chief nurse officer of that particular service/division/department.

2. **Council responsibility:** With the executive officer and the elected leaders of the councils, the executive/coordinating council takes form and becomes the decision-making body that integrates the organizational system. It does not usurp or remove responsibilities or accountabilities from the governing councils or from the unit-level councils. The executive/coordinating council is responsible for:

- Integration: This is a fundamental responsibility of this group. In fact, the executive council has no accountability *except* the responsibilities designated to it by the governing councils. It focuses on integration, conflict resolution, goal setting, operations, and bylaws.

- Conflict resolution: Between and among councils, between staff and councils, and between management and councils, the council resolves conflict in the organization as a whole.

- Goal setting: The council sets the goals and objectives for the division, reviews the budget, and settles those issues that are in question or need to be clarified to ensure that the set direction moves forward. It sees that the structure and relationships in the organizational system operate effectively. The success of the system is dependent on the integration, coordination, and facilitation of its various functions.

- Bylaws: This group is responsible for the construction of the bylaws (see Appendixes 4, 5, and 6). They form, manage, control, adapt, and change the bylaws as needed. Change may come from anywhere in the organization. However, that change must be submitted to this elected and appointed coordinating council to determine that it does not in some way harm the integrity of the organization. After, the change recommendation can be submitted to the staff council as a whole in general session at the annual meeting for inclusion in the bylaws revision and review. The bylaws then take form and can be adjusted legitimately and equitably without threatening the integrity of the organizational system. From this, leadership and direction for development of the governance process evolves.

3. **Leadership and governance:** Leadership emerges from all the places in the organizational system. Direct-care nurse leadership is essential to the successful implementation of shared governance. The leadership role of the manager, too, is critical. This role changes dramatically in the terms of behavior modification, development, and exercising the management role as shared governance processes create new behaviors essential to success in the new structural process model.

Importance of the manager

1. **Developmental processes** occur at different rates in different places but with the same outcomes. Empowered organizations cannot be managed in the same way as traditional organizations.

As direct-care nurses mature in their professional behaviors and exercise ownership and accountability, those new behaviors will impact the role of the manager. Clearly, managers in the organizational system are needed—it is a myth to assume that the management process disappears in empowerment processes. The role evolves into exemplified, servant leadership due to the resource nature of the role.

2. **New characteristics of the role** are broader. In the traditional definition of the role, the manager was the planner, leader, organizer, and controller of the system. The empowering manager will develop other characteristics (coordinator, facilitator, integrator), with the ability to pull those pieces together and to exemplify those roles in a shared decision-making model. This is critical to the manager's success in applying the new role and exercising it to make a difference in the resources available for the direct-care nurse decision-makers.

Unit-level councils in shared governance

In the midst of the shared governance process, the unit-level councils must be well established. Shared governance cannot make a difference if the units do not establish their own councils representing their own culture and designed in a way that fulfills their own needs and concerns in the governing councils. The only caveat for this process is that the units fulfill the principles directed for them by the governance councils and provided for them in the organizational structure. Using these principles and applying them to the unit councils will ensure that there will be organizational consistency and that the organization as a whole will implement shared governance successfully.

In the final analysis, it is important to know that shared governance is not the property of any individual, department, division, or discipline. It is a universal organizational management process model, a way of working together to accomplish goals and objectives that invests all the participants in shared decision-making, partnership, equity, accountability, and ownership. It is a practical approach for reshaping and transforming professional nursing practice at the point of service.

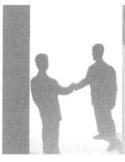

BUILDING THE UNIT-LEVEL PRACTICE COUNCIL FOR IMPLEMENTING SHARED GOVERNANCE AT POINT OF CARE

LEARNING OBJECTIVES

After reading this chapter, the participant should be able to:

- Describe the importance of a unit-level council

- List three strategies to help nurses accept change when establishing and building a unit council

- Identify the first three steps in building a unit-level practice council

Never tell people how to do things. Tell them what to do and they will surprise you with their ingenuity.

– George S. Patton

Why Is a Unit-Level Council So Important?

The unit council is the core structure for nursing shared governance. Unit-level shared governance provides a critical forum to give all direct-care nurses assigned to a particular unit an opportunity to participate in shared decisional processes and outcomes specific to the needs and activities of that unit. Although all staff of all levels may participate, unit councils are led and managed by the direct-care professional nurse. Members of the unit council identify, explore, and resolve issues, questions, ideas, and concerns related to professional nursing practice, quality, competency, education, and the work environment. But first, they must ask themselves some difficult questions, such as:

- What is my role in shared governance?

- How do I view the nursing environment, nursing leadership, interprofessional partnerships,

interdisciplinary teams, the professional practice model, and patient care
delivery systems?

- What do I want to contribute at the unit level? At the department/division level? At the
  organization level? At the community level?

- What support is available for the additional time needed to participate equitably in shared
  governance at the varied levels of responsibility and accountability?

- What resources and skills do I need to be successful in my professional role on this unit? In
  this organization?

Once they have explored their own possible contributions and ideas about shared governance, members of
the unit council should challenge themselves with the following questions as they move forward to help
build and/or expand the unit council:

1. **Are we doing it right?**

   - Are direct-care nurses leading the unit council?

   - Is the nurse manager/supervisor supportive of staff participating in the unit council and
     related/assigned activities?

   - Are human, material, and fiscal resources (e.g., time, staffing, and supplies) available for the
     work of the unit council?

   - Is nurse participation in the unit council by invitation or mandated?

   - Is there a formal structure for holding meetings and reporting outcomes?

2. **Are we doing the right thing well?**

   - Are managers, nurses, and staff appropriately involved in the unit council when needed?

   - Is the agenda appropriate and manageable for the time allocated for the unit council meeting?

   - Is there a facilitator to help participants achieve the desired outcomes and meeting objectives?

- Is the unit meeting coordinated well enough to ensure continuity and participation by members while others manage patient care?

- Are meetings and activities (i.e., quality dashboards, safety, contributions to practice policies, evidence-based nursing practice, point-of-care research) managed in an efficient manner with due consideration given to allocation of resources to engage in shared decision-making and shared leadership at point of care and to address issues related to practice, quality, and competence?

3. **Do job descriptions and functional statements for registered nurses reflect the language of shared governance** related to professional nursing practice, autonomy, ownership, equity, partnership, responsibility and accountability, authority, quality, and competency?

Dealing With Change

Building the unit-level practice council for implementing shared governance at point of care is about change—how do we make change painless?

> Change has a considerable psychological impact on the human mind.
> To the fearful it is threatening because it means that things may get worse.
> To the hopeful it is encouraging because things may get better.
> To the confident it is inspiring because the challenge exists to make things better.
>
> — *King Whitney, Jr.*

Changing technology, increasing acuities, patients and families who are more knowledgeable about healthcare, and emerging paradigm shifts … Change is our only constant. Nurses must embrace new skills, take more professional risks, and reach further than ever before. What an exciting time to be a nurse.

Yet nobody actually *likes* change. New technologies and processes, skills, and professional demands seem costly, risky, frighteningly complicated, and too time-consuming to learn. The resulting stress can make nurses feel increasingly overwhelmed and overworked. Change occurs so quickly that unfreezing from past behaviors is no longer possible before new demands consume our attention. There is rarely time to become comfortable with new information before it is being replaced with even newer ideas, processes, and concepts with a promise of higher quality and lower cost. The answer: partnerships and strategies to help nurses accept change and realize future possibilities.

Change may not be an option, but how to engage in it is open to negotiation and does not have to be painful (Schoemer, 2009):

- Begin with the right attitude

- Let your confidence show

- Be autonomous in practice and presence

- Be an expert learner

- Be solution-oriented

- Speak up

- Create and innovate

- Let integrity rule

- Communicate and relate

- Strike a balance between work and play

- Become a teacher/preceptor/coach/mentor

- Be a student of the "business" of healthcare

- Be flexibly adaptive

- Be a servant leader, formally and informally

Servant (Transformational) Leadership

Nurses understand and practice servant leadership at every level of care—it begins with a desire to serve others. Such service has the power to transform the lives of those who serve and those who are served.

It builds relationships with meaning, purpose, and respect. It is unique to the one who has the ability to serve and lead. Power is not coercive. It is used to create opportunity and alternatives so that others may choose and build autonomy.

Transactional leaders (those who use a power model of leadership, sometimes referred to as *micromanagers*) are more evident in most healthcare organizations at all levels. They are not problematic to the success of an organization and are often good, intelligent, vital people who manage tasks, events, programs, resources, and technology quite well. Problems arise when they try to manage rather than lead people. Frequently, positional power or authority is used to coerce, intimidate, or control staff rather than engage them. The relationship frequently has a parent-child feel to it.

Transforming (servant) leaders are more complex and potent than other leaders. This leader recognizes an existing need or demand and then looks beyond it to motive and greater need (i.e., Maslow's hierarchy), and engages the whole person. The result is a relationship of mutual trust, inspiration, respect, and potential that elevates staff to servant leaders. Such leaders are transformative.

A *servant leader*, then, is simply a leader intent on serving others, one who loves people and wants to help them. Because servant leadership is first and foremost an act of service, it transforms two internal and two external domains of the one who would lead:

- Internal

    - Heart—motivations: self-serving (egocentric) vs. serving others

    - Head—leadership point of view

- External

    - Hands—public leadership behaviors

    - Habits—habits as by others

Leadership is about moving from a self-serving heart to a serving one. True leadership is about what we give, rather than what we get (Blanchard & Hodges, 2003; Greenleaf, 1991, 2008; Nightingale, 1992).

When nurses approach shared governance with the same genuineness they employ in patient care, they will find these transformative qualities in their own leadership and expressed in the collaborative relationships they build. A unit council is not another work group. It is a unique structure for nurses to practice their profession through shared decisional processes and transformational, servant leadership.

Building Relationships: Interprofessional and Interdisciplinary Teams

Nurses do not work in silos. Healthcare organizations are incredibly complex macrosystems. Although unit councils operate at the microsystem level, it is important for direct-care nurses and staff working at point of service to think about the "big picture" when building relationships.

The pharmacy staff at one facility were becoming overwhelmed with the growing number of demands and stat orders from a particular medical-surgical nursing unit. Some nurses were adding "stat" to requests to expedite their orders rather than because of actual need. After several attempts to speak to the behaviors and explain the escalating problems they caused in the pharmacy, the chief of pharmacy services asked to attend a unit council meeting. He never mentioned the tension among staff members or how busy his own team was, though. Instead, during the council meeting, he invited the nurses to tour the pharmacy after lunch and arranged for them to see their new technology and services.

They did—and arrived at the busiest, most chaotic time of the day. Machines shouted. Orders flew. Telephones shrieked. Patients demanded. The pharmacy staff took it all with grace (mostly), dignity, and a herculean effort to respond to every request, shout, shriek, and demand. The nurses watched in awe and left with greater respect for the pharmacy staff's workload. Thanking the chief, the nurses returned to their units, scheduled a special council meeting with a representative from the pharmacy to participate in their discussion, and tackled the problem. Together, they collaborated on new guidelines for how the nurses could manage pharmacy orders more efficiently and what pharmacy staff could contribute equitably. The relationships they built continue to thrive and grow.

See Figure 4.1 for an example of a unit-level microsystem.

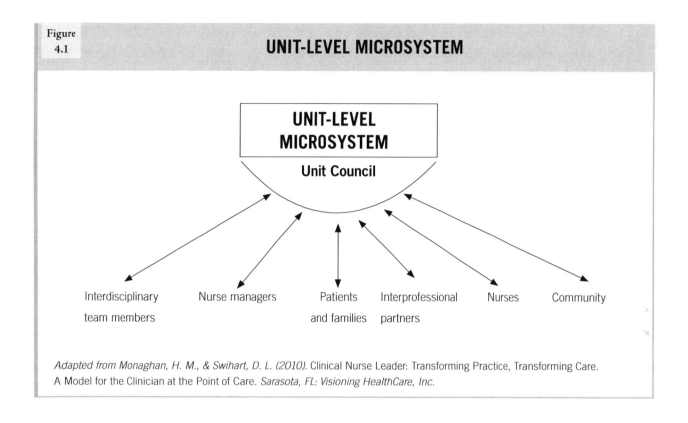

Figure 4.1

UNIT-LEVEL MICROSYSTEM

UNIT-LEVEL MICROSYSTEM

Unit Council

Interdisciplinary team members Nurse managers Patients and families Interprofessional partners Nurses Community

Adapted from Monaghan, H. M., & Swihart, D. L. (2010). Clinical Nurse Leader: Transforming Practice, Transforming Care. A Model for the Clinician at the Point of Care. *Sarasota, FL: Visioning HealthCare, Inc.*

The unit council offers an opportunity for nurses to take control of their own practice; to engage with interdisciplinary team members, interprofessional partners, leadership, patients and families, and guests from other communities of practice and points of service; and to build the relationships essential to successful patient care outcomes. When selecting tools, setting up a unit council, and determining what to add to the agenda, nurses include important linkages with:

- Interprofessional partners (physicians, nurses, pharmacists)

- Other interdisciplinary team members (e.g., managers/supervisors, clinical nurse leaders, dietitians, pharmacy representatives, advanced practice nurses, educators and staff development specialists, social workers, chaplains, environmental services)

- Central governance councils

- Organization and service line committees

◆ Communities of practice (i.e., those who share a profession and engage in a process of collective learning through interaction and shared decision-making)

◆ Communities of service (engagement with and service to members of local communities [i.e., a unit council that provides CPR training to local school nurses as a community/public service each year])

With continuous change inherent in the work we do, keeping pace with those changes and making appropriate adjustments in our approach to engaging in shared governance are a constant challenge. Recognizing this, we would like to take a fresh look at unit councils here and offer some sample tools and techniques to help guide implementation and improvements in establishing a strong structure and shared decisional processes.

The tools and templates included in this book and available with the downloadable resources were developed and/or selected in response to many of the requests received over the past five years from nurses engaged in shared governance at the unit level. It is hoped they will add value and reduce the amount of time and effort required to establish or advance your councils. (See the list of figures and tools page for a complete listing of sample tools that are available for download on the downloadable resources page. You can also find an expanded bibliography that presents additional readings and research on shared governance.)

Building the Structure for Unit-Level Practice Councils (The Microsystem Level of Shared Governance)

Step 1. Select a structure for designing/steering the development of a model for unit councils

Establish a design team or steering committee of staff members to develop the structures and guiding principles for unit-level councils in nursing service. Because this structure is nurse-driven, the majority of team members should be direct-care nurses with input from nurse managers and the executive nurse. This team develops the initial model and infrastructure of unit-level councils and provides tools to help nurses implement the templates at point of service. Unit teams will then further develop their councils according to their own work and goals.

Select a chair for the design team. If this person is a direct-care nurse, a cochair might be a nurse manager to provide guidance, resources, and boundaries as appropriate as the work evolves.

Select a liaison or facilitator for the design team. This person facilitates communication within nursing service, among the nursing staff as the unit councils are being formed, and as a contact person for the governing councils and nurse leaders. Although not required, a liaison/facilitator helps free up the other members of the design team or steering committee to do the work of developing the unit council structures, processes, and targeted outcomes. Once the unit councils are established, a facilitator can continue to monitor and oversee long-term unit projects.

Note: Once a person commits to working on the design team or steering committee, attendance and participation are *not* optional. Make sure nurse managers and supervisors are informed of scheduled meetings and assigned duties related to the work of the design team/steering committee to better facilitate staff involvement.

List the key drivers for unit councils (e.g., professional practice, quality and safety, competency and professional excellence, evidence-based nursing practice and research, peer review, best practices, collaborative relationships, awards and recognition, operations), as distinguished from accountabilities for shared decision-making and collaborations of nurse leaders and direct-care nurses (Haag-Heitman & George, 2010; Porter-O'Grady, 2009a, 2009b, 2009c), including:

- Nurse leaders (i.e., managers/supervisors):

    - Administrative operations and resources (human, material, fiscal)

    - Work environment/structure to facilitate autonomy and professionalism

    - Organization/macrosystem and department/mesosystem linkages

    - Rewards and recognitions related to performance appraisals/evaluations

    - Nursing strategic planning

- Direct-care nurses:

  - Unit council and practice operations

  - Standards of practice (specialty and clinical competencies; professional practice models)

  - Care delivery systems

  - Professional development (clinical and academic activities; orientation, preceptorships and mentorships, continuing education, certifications)

  - Quality improvement (evidence-based practice, research, quality outcomes)

  - Peer review (competency, performance evaluations, 360-degree assessments, feedback)

  - Interdisciplinary team relationships

  - Interprofessional partnerships

  - Nursing strategic planning

Step 2. Develop the unit council bylaws or charter

Discuss the key drivers identified and select a framework for the operations and management of the unit council, usually bylaws or a charter (see Appendix 4, sample unit-level bylaws, and Appendix 8, sample unit-level charter). Simple guiding principles generally are not strong enough to establish the unit council as a formal structure for shared governance. Bylaws and/or charters, documents describing the formal organization and operations of the unit council and membership, emphasize the importance of the councils and their professional activities.

Develop a generic set of unit council bylaws or a charter with formal descriptions for all levels of participation, responsibilities, and accountabilities:

- Membership (nominations, term limits, commitment, dismissal from service)

- Meetings/timelines (how often and for how long; set calendar for at least a year at a time)

                                                           SHARED GOVERNANCE, SECOND EDITION

- Communications (respectful, open, honest, focused); describe how communications will:

    - Be disseminated among unit-level staff on all shifts and off-tours (e.g., weekends and holidays)

    - Flow within and among units and other practice settings (e.g., e-mail, bulletin boards, Share-Point site, newsletters [i.e., *Hospice Unit Council Newsletter*], staff meetings)

    - Flow between/among governing (central) councils (see Appendix 7, sample nursing governance council action request form; Appendix 9, sample nursing communication policy; Appendix 10, sample communication flow chart; Appendix 11, sample coordinating council attendance form; and Appendix 12, sample coordinating council agenda/minutes template)

- Responsibilities and accountabilities:

    - Direct-care nurses

    - Nursing leadership

    - Clinical nurse leaders (quality systems and performance measures at point of care)

    - Clinical educators and staff development specialists

    - Advanced practice nurses

    - Interdisciplinary team members (when invited to a meeting)

Step 3. Determine what happens in a unit-level practice council meeting

Agenda and minutes (see Appendix 29, sample unit council agenda/minutes template; Appendix 13, sample unit council minutes with notes; and Appendix 14, sample sign-in form)

Topics for discussion and decision-making (related to practice, quality, and competence) include:

- Clinical practice (grounded in evidence-based practice and practice-based evidence)

- Participatory/self-scheduling

- Time management (i.e., organization, prioritization, and delegation)

+ Quality management systems and performance measures (i.e., the plan, do, check, act process)

+ Professional development and education (see Appendix 15, a guideline for unit councils: performance improvement at the unit level)

+ Peer review (professional/institutional, performance, and competency; see Appendix 16, sample peer evaluation for charge nurses)

+ Research and evidence-based nursing practice at point of care

+ Journal club (articles, action plans, and after-action reviews; see Appendix 17, a guide to unit-level journal clubs; and Appendix 18, sample after-action review form)

+ Nursing administration and leadership (role of manager in unit-level practice council meetings)

+ Financial stewardship at point of care and improved fiscal outcomes

+ Contributing to strategic plans (see Appendix 19, unit level strategic planning with the strengths, weaknesses, opportunities, and threats [SWOT] template; and Appendix 20, sample nursing strategic planning tool)

Sample tools to help unit councils with discussion and decision-making include:

+ Unit council worksheet (see Appendix 3) to help identify specific topics related to categories of shared decisional opportunities

+ Unit council discussion planner (see Appendix 21) to help focus discussions for projects, expectations, decisions, actions, reporting of outcomes, and follow-up related to topics/events under discussion

+ Unit council shared decision-making tool (see Appendix 22) to guide processes for shared decision-making within the shared governance structures and build more effective teams

Example of the flow of a unit council meeting:

+ Welcome attendees and make introductions (especially of guests)—make sure everyone has signed in (see Appendix 14, sample unit council sign-in form)

- Review minutes from previous unit council meeting and approve or approve with corrections

- Nurse manager's visit (usually five to 10 minutes)

- *Note:* Do not confuse unit council meetings with staff meetings. They each have very different purposes and expected outcomes. Many units have one of the following constructs:

  - A staff meeting that is separate from the unit council meeting (different time, different day).

  - The nurse manager attends the unit council meeting for about five to 10 minutes to offer information or respond to questions from council attendees. Sometimes, the nurse manager's visit occurs at the end of a unit council meeting.

  - The staff meeting generally belongs to the nurse manager or designee.

  - The unit-council meetings belong to the direct-care nurses.

- Presentations/discussions by guests, if present (e.g., infection control nurse, representative from a central council requested to bring more information/guidance, dietitian, research nurse)

- Address new business (e.g., topic identified and discussed, assignments given, deadlines set)

- Address old business (e.g., previous topics and assignments discussed, follow-up, deadlines met)

- Recommendations for next agenda

- Adjournment

- Report of meeting minutes completed and disseminated to nurse manager and all unit staff:

  - After-action reviews and activities (e.g., changing practice, building competency, precepting and mentoring, advancing improvements in quality, safety, and efficiency; see Appendix 18, sample after action review form, and Appendix 23, sample unit quarterly report form)

  - Celebrations (celebrating coworkers and team members [i.e., graduations, certifications, ideas, promotions and advancements, accomplishments, best practices, birthdays, anniversaries, etc.])

Step 4. Explore ways to change practice and influence organizational outcomes through strategic planning and actions

Shared governance, especially when first implemented, is a major change in an organization. Therefore, nurses need to orchestrate the change in the most meaningful way possible for all members actively and passively engaged in the process. All levels of nurses participate in developing the nursing service strategic plan, the key to a successful implementation. They develop an organizing framework, a measurement tool, timeline, and list of accountabilities assigned to each of the central governance councils and the unit-level councils (see Appendix 20, sample nursing strategic planning tool). The nurse executive provides the organizational strategic plan to ensure alignment of the nursing service and unit-level plans with the organization's overarching mission, vision, key drivers, and strategic goals (Haag-Heitman & George, 2010).

Nursing strategic planning begins at the unit level and involves all levels of nurses in the process. It is a road map for ensuring leadership and staff are aligned and going in the right direction, and a process for identifying strategies and making decisions on allocating unit resources to achieve specific outcomes around practice, quality, and competency.

> The difference between where we are and where we want to be is what we do.
>
> – *Author Unknown*

Strategic planning helps leadership and staff members determine where a unit (department and/or organization) is going over the next year or longer, usually three to five years. To do this, the unit council needs to know exactly where it is currently, then decide where it wants to go and how it will get there. Begin by conducting an environmental scan, a process for collecting data to answer questions about the present and future of the unit, department, and organization using such tools as surveys, questionnaires, focus groups, and open forums to:

+ Develop a common perception

+ Identify strengths, weaknesses, trends, and conditions

+ Draw on internal and external information

Strategic planning produces ideas and actions. Various techniques can be used in strategic planning, including SWOT analysis. SWOT analysis is useful in decision-making for multiple situations and activities, for identifying ideas and seeing how they relate to each other (see Appendix 19, sample unit-level strategic planning with SWOT template). These headings provide a good framework for reviewing strategy, position, ideas, and direction of a unit council. It also works well in brainstorming meetings and team building exercises. (For more information and many free tools for implementing this approach to problem solving and strategic planning, go to SWOT analysis method and examples, with free SWOT template at *www.businessballs.com*.) Describe the situation and set goals and objectives/outcomes:

- Conduct a SWOT analysis based on the identified goals

- Establish actions and/or processes needed to achieve these goals

- Implement agreed-on actions, processes, changes in practice, etc., to operationalize the plan

- Monitor and get feedback from responsible person(s)

- Recognize benchmarks and deadlines when met

- Communicate changes made in practice, improvements in safety and patient care, and other achievements related to outcomes of strategic planning

- Evaluate and update strategic plans; identify methods for periodic review, evaluation, and revision to ensure plans and actions are aligned and on track

The primary purpose for strategic plans is action, strategies translated into day-to-day projects and tasks required to achieve the plan. One way to keep individual workloads at a manageable level is to delegate different topics to ad hoc teams (e.g., a journal club, a quality improvement team, a policies and procedures work group). The goals of unit strategic planning must fit with the department/division and organization strategic plans. Examples of questions to consider when involved in strategic planning must look at governance and equity:

- Strategic planning around governance:

    - What existing policies, procedures, and/or statutes encourage or inhibit the strategic planning at the unit level?

- How will the introduction of strategic planning affect the way the unit works?

- How will the unit council participants adjust to make the best use of strategic planning and implementation?

- How can the strategic plan be used to improve all aspects of the unit council's operation?

- How will staff and leadership know if the strategic plan's objectives have been met?

- How will decisions about resources, schedules, practice, competencies, and patient safety and care be made?

- Will these decisions be part of the larger strategic plans for the department/division or organization?

+ Strategic planning around equity:

- How can strategic planning and implementation of changes benefit all staff?

- How will staff on all shifts and those unable to participate in strategic planning benefit from the changes?

- How can strategic planning benefit direct-care nurses?

- How can strategic planning benefit resistant or disengaged staff, or those who are not performing well?

When developing strategies, analyze the unit and its environment as it is presently and how it may develop in the future. The final SWOT analysis helps staff identify multiple ideas, questions, and issues, and agree on those ideas relatively quickly. The outcomes form the consensus on themes or ideas generated by the unit council, department, or organization. This is best achieved when nurses:

+ Participate in unit-level strategic planning (see Appendix 24, unit council strategic planning tool)

+ Participate in service-level (department/division) strategic planning (see Appendix 20, nursing strategic planning tool)

+ Participate in organization-level strategic planning

The analysis has to be executed at an internal level as well as an external level to identify all opportunities and threats of the external environment as well as the strengths and weaknesses of the unit, the department, and the organization. Once the strategic plan is in place, it must be communicated.

Collaborate and communicate with all stakeholder groups. Engage all unit staff, interdisciplinary team members, and interprofessional partners in the strategic plan and outcomes. When others are engaged, they have an opportunity to participate and provide input.

Step 5. Troubleshooting obstacles and meeting challenges to shared governance at the point of care

> When we are no longer able to change a situation, we are challenged to change ourselves.
>
> —*Victor Frankl*

Meeting challenges at the point of care (i.e., engagement, disengagement, resistance):

- **Petulant participants** (Hess, n.d.). Nurse managers and charge nurses communicate to all staff that shared governance and the activities in the unit council are not optional. Even then, some people will resist. It is important to engage them, too:

  – Pull everyone in through education about what shared governance is and what it can do for their practice; emphasize the importance the organization ascribes to the shared governance program and activities; eliminate nonparticipation as an option

  – Assess and develop direct-care nurses' knowledge and experience in leading and participating in shared decisional processes; nurses may have been managed (often micromanaged) for so long they withdraw, having become comfortable with tasked assignments, and may fear the added responsibility and accountability inherent in shared governance; provide education, mentoring, and opportunities for them to participate fully in shared governance

  – Organize an involvement-friendly environment that is as easy as possible for all staff who are interested in doing so to attend meetings; shift focus from the individual to the group; praise the enthusiasm of participants; build a sense of commitment and ownership

– Shared governance is not appropriate for every healthcare organization and not right for every nurse; true detractors can make one of three choices: (1) refuse to participate and accept decisions from the group; (2) participate informally in limited activities without attending formal meetings; or (3) refuse to participate on any level and, eventually, move on to find a better fit elsewhere

– Make sure everyone has the job- and role-appropriate skills needed for shared governance; do not confuse expertise with position or role

– Set a realistic time frame for achieving goals; give staff time, information, and encouragement—not everyone joins in at the same rate or time; as changes are made, benchmark and chart progress

* **Troublesome managers.** These are often individuals placed in positions of leadership without sufficient orientation or training to prepare them for their roles, especially in areas of shared governance, transformational leadership, crucial conversations, and managing workplace complexities.

– Many managers are experienced in transactional leadership, often grounded in how they were managed early in their own careers and what they draw on when placed in leadership roles: provide education and mentoring in transformational leadership skills.

– Frequently, individuals were promoted into nurse manager positions and nurse leader roles because of their clinical expertise, not their skills in either management or leadership: educate, mentor, and encourage them in building knowledge, skill, and confidence.

– Shared governance may elicit fear (i.e., false evidence appearing real) in managers asked to delegate tasks to staff that they had always considered "their" job: engage them in new roles, facilitate letting go of legacy systems, help them develop new skills.

– Some nurse managers refuse to adapt and engage in shared governance—they will not support their staff in transitioning into autonomous professional practice or align themselves with the direction of the organization in implementing shared governance. In such cases, the nurse executive may set a realistic time frame and participation goals for these nurse managers to achieve. Managers do not have the same gift of time as staff to engage. As leaders, they must be among the first on board with shared governance or it will not occur at point of care or organizationally.

- Shared governance needs to be built into the nursing service strategic plan with supporting education, resources, and accountabilities for nurse managers. Nurse managers are critical to the success of shared governance. They:

  ○ Establish a work environment to support shared governance

  ○ Set expectations of staff participation in unit councils, committees, and central councils

  ○ Facilitate staff readiness to change, adapt, and evaluate their own practice, quality, competency, and to engage in participatory scheduling and peer reviews

  ○ Manage staffing patterns and resources to support staff involvement in unit council

- **Hesitant participants.** Find the underlying cause that holds them back and address it. The following examples of concerns by many direct-care nurses about engaging in shared governance activities were taken from multiple nurse satisfaction surveys and have been reported in the literature since the first edition of this book was published in 2006:

  - Too much responsibility and accountability but not enough authority

  - Not enough control over schedules

  - A perceived gap (communication and interaction) between administration and nursing

  - Nurse manager does not support shared governance or a unit council

  - Not enough opportunities for advancement or education

  - Lack of autonomy

  - Lack of respect and/or collegiality from interprofessional partners

  - Not enough opportunity for staff to participate in administrative decision-making processes

  - Little or no voice in the planning of unit policies and procedures, determining unit-based competencies, or managing their own performance measures and/or outcomes

    – Little or no time/resources given to participate in decision-making processes

    – Nursing administrators do not consult with staff on daily problems/procedures at point of care

Avoid isolating unit councils. Make sure the structures and lines of communication are established before or during the establishment of unit-level councils. Some organizations will set up a pilot council to see how it functions prior to setting up the entire shared governance infrastructure. Although this approach may have some success, it can cause an imbalance or disconnect between the earlier established council and those that follow (i.e., when a microsystem becomes self-sufficient and autonomous without interacting with other central or unit councils, interdisciplinary teams, or external stakeholders, it can lead to isolation and an inability to fit readily back into the whole of the organization's shared governance macrosystem or even nursing service's mesosystem).

Facilitate time for regularly scheduled unit council meetings. The needs of direct-care nurses and staff to provide safe, quality patient care always takes precedence. This means meetings may need to be shortened or held by e-mail, for example, to continue the operations of the unit council.

Direct-care nurses need time away from the unit and patient care assignments to work on projects and assignments for the unit council (or a committee or central council) to help advance practice at point of care, do research, or improve staff competencies. Nurse managers and charge nurses are critical in helping nurses do the important work of the unit council and still meet the patient care needs of often exceedingly busy units.

Gaining buy-in from the other staff and direct-care nurses. Many direct-care nurses have only a vague idea of what council or committee members do at meetings or during time away from the unit. To gain buy-in, do the following:

+ Communication is key. Share minutes and information about projects with staff. Invite them to contribute their own thoughts and talents to completing assignments.

+ Negotiate schedules to allow equitable time for everyone to have special consideration of their requests whenever possible.

- One organization hired resource nurses to cover unit patient care assignments while regular staff participated in their shared governance meetings and activities.

- Develop subcommittees or task groups/forces to engage all staff members, interdisciplinary team members, and even patients and families (e.g., surveys, interviews) in projects to improve care at point of service through unit councils.

- Share successes and celebrations, even small ones, with the entire staff.

Measuring the benefits and success of unit councils and shared governance models at point of care:

- Examine data collected from chart reviews, surveys, and performance measures

- Collect and analyze unit data

- Use dashboards or scorecards to display data; communicate data findings and changes to practice related to those findings in unit council meetings

- Identify changes in practice related to data collected (e.g., Index for Professional Nursing Governance scores, patient satisfaction, RN satisfaction, nursing quality indicators)

- Benchmark and measure effectiveness of unit programs based on data

- Provide concrete feedback to staff for their competencies and clinical practice

- Report findings and applications to practice to all direct-care nurses and other staff

Evaluating and restructuring the unit council may be necessary whenever the current structure is no longer effective; there are significant changes in staffing mix, patient populations, or nurse leadership; or organizational redesign causes physical changes in the unit infrastructure (i.e., merging two units and reducing the number of direct-care nurses working on the newly reconfigured unit). Follow these steps:

- *Build an effective team.* The role of nurses and teams in shared governance is multifaceted and covers a wide range of activities. Building an effective team is key to building and managing professional, interdisciplinary teams at point of care:

    - Assess current team functioning

– Discuss potential positive and negative outcomes for implementing shared governance at the unit level and what this means to the team:

○ Implementing and/or advancing shared governance will reduce the negative outcomes (e.g., increased time and effort needed to establish and participate in shared decisional processes) and maintain or increase positive outcomes (i.e., shared leadership) of how the team is currently functioning in terms of practice, quality, and competency

○ What has to be done differently to engage in shared governance

○ How to best support and engage in shared governance:

▪ To reduce negative or increase positive consequences

▪ To engage in the new behaviors

▪ To develop the characteristics of an effective unit team

Characteristics of an effective unit team

If any of the following characteristics do not make sense to the team or fit the unique tasks, resources, and organization policies/procedures relevant to the responsibilities and accountabilities of each member of the team according to his or her scope of practice and/or job description, the team will address the inconsistencies to build a more effective team. This is essential if team members are to participate in shared decision-making equitably.

Note: Not all decisions are shared. At times, managers/supervisors may have to direct or assign a task or activity or point out a boundary that cannot be breached organizationally. At such times, these are decisions already made by others and are only for information and/or compliance by the employee. However, this information may also bear on other decisions by the unit council and/or team members and is important to building an effective unit team.

Leadership:

• Unit council chair/designated leader accepts responsibility but does not dominate team

• Leadership may shift, depending on the issue—servant/transformational leadership evidenced

• It is not about control but how to get the job done

- Decisions that cannot be resolved at unit level are directed to the central (governance) council(s) as appropriate (see Appendix 7, sample nursing governance council action request form)

- Nurse managers usually take an advisory role and support the processes of shared decision-making through proactive scheduling and communication with staff, charge nurses, and unit council leadership

- Charge nurses usually contribute by supporting initiatives on the unit, communicating with nurse manager, staff, and unit council members, facilitating council attendance, and managing resistance and change

Work environment:

- Nurse managers help set the climate for unit-level shared governance

- Support shared governance at point of care

- Combination of formal and informal activities

- Mutually respectful interactions among physicians, nurses, and other team members

- Professional, autonomous environment of care

- People are interested and engaged

Clarity and acceptance of tasks and goals:

- Clear, understood, and generally accepted

- Participative, not autocratically directed or assigned without staff input

- Everyone participates

- Everyone knows what they are supposed to do or not do

- Clear assignments are made and accepted

- Nurse managers ensure staff attendance, participation, and accountability by nurses and staff involved in the unit council and other councils and committees

- Monitor activities and progress; report progress, benchmarks, deadlines, and outcomes as they occur (see Appendix 25, sample activities in progress form)

- Nurse managers and staff participate in strategic planning through unit councils and department/division and organization committees

- If there are questions, a contact person(s) is available

Decisions:

- Clear and determined in a way that team members are in consensus and willing to support them (see Appendix 22, sample unit council shared decision-making tool)

- Persons who oppose the decision will speak up or notify the unit council chair or other(s), as appropriate depending on the reason for the disagreement

- Use disagreements to explore other options, concerns, or possible consequences to ensure the final decision is the best one

- If disagreements are outside of issues related to practice, quality, competency, unit operations, or boundaries (i.e., personnel issues), nurse managers may advise/guide unit councils how to best proceed

- If immediate disagreements cannot be resolved, the team leader may need to table the discussion/decision until further information/support can be obtained

Feedback:

- Active listening with reflective feedback

- Constructive, consistent, clear

- Peer reviews: process done consistently and according to policy (see Appendix 16, sample peer evaluation for charge nurses)

- Individually: as needed—there should be no surprises or bundled complaints

- Unit: provide a report of activities at least quarterly to nurse manager and all unit staff (see Appendix 23, sample unit quarterly report form)

- Provide ongoing reports to nurse managers at interdisciplinary team meetings, nursing assemblies, nursing town hall meetings, and at central (governance) council meetings when appropriate (i.e., improvements in performance measures and nursing quality indicators reported to the central nursing governance quality council)

Advocacy:

- Become comfortable with risk management and confronting team members with potential problems that can result in medical errors and impact nurse and patient safety

- Creatively problem solve and resolve/manage conflict (see Appendix 26, sample conflict resolution worksheet)

- Accept responsibility for mistakes and near misses and intervene to maintain/reestablish nurse and patient safety

- Provide regular in-services and support for ethical practice among healthcare providers

- Recognize and protect (see Appendix 27, nurses' bill of rights in shared governance)

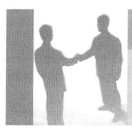

IMPLEMENTING SHARED GOVERNANCE AT THE ORGANIZATION LEVEL

After reading this chapter, the participant should be able to:

- Discuss the roles of the following stakeholders: leadership, union representatives, community members, nurses, and patients

- Describe how shared governance can be an integrating structure in healthcare organizations under nursing's leadership

No significant learning occurs without a significant relationship.

– James Comer, MD

The Roles of the Stakeholders

A consortium of stakeholders is needed to participate in shared governance for it to succeed: researchers, administrators, nurse executives, direct-care nurses, interdisciplinary team members, patients, and community members. Their roles are as diverse and interrelated as their expertise, experiences, and education. Four such stakeholders, or partners, include leadership, union representatives, community members, and patients.

Leadership partners in shared governance

Shared governance helps those in leadership positions—administrators, nurse executives, nurse managers, supervisors—step back from many tasks and decisions about practice, quality, and competency direct-care nurses are more than qualified to make. Nurse leaders provide a professional practice environment that supports and facilitates direct-care nurse autonomy.

Union partners in shared governance

Although a complex system with many guidelines and regulations, the simplified purpose of the union in most healthcare organizations is two-fold:

1. Collective bargaining to help nurses gain control over their practice and accomplish professional and economic goals, objectives, and outcomes

2. Protection from demanding and/or unfair management standards that threaten the quality of nursing care or negatively impact the professional practice environment (e.g., unsafe or ineffective staffing ratios, mandatory overtime, and unsafe or hostile work environments, among others)

Even though both collective bargaining and shared governance are about giving nurses a voice in decision-making in ways that impact practice at the point of service and organizationwide, shared governance is not collective bargaining. Shared governance is a shared decision-making process.

The goal in shared governance is to integrate collaborative practice into the professional practice environment through shared decision-making. By partnering with the union representatives in the healthcare organization from the beginning of implementation, the interdisciplinary team members can communicate this intent and address concerns and issues as they arise, thereby increasing understanding and reducing or eliminating the confrontation that sometimes occurs in such discussions (Porter-O'Grady, 2004).

Community partners in shared governance

Nurses engaged in shared governance partner with members of their communities in activities that reflect positively on the organization and nursing service. They share in the decision-making around which activities to support and to offer. Community collaborations include those with direct-care nurses participating in outreach programs, such as:

+   Offering a CPR day for community members each year

+   Presenting a health fair annually with direct-care nurses negotiating the vendors and activities for various patient populations from the community and their families (e.g., prostate cancer screenings, smoking cessation programs, and disaster preparedness activities)

+   Obtaining affiliations with local universities and colleges for nurses to continue their academic educations on hospital grounds

- Allocating and using appropriate resources to support various projects (e.g., a junior internship program that brings high school students into the organization during the summer and teaches them how to communicate with patients)

Patients as partners in shared governance

Patients today are very knowledgeable and unwilling to be directed in their treatment plans. They want a voice in what treatment approaches will be implemented, which medications they will take, and even where they will be hospitalized. Shared governance is an integrating structure (Porter-O'Grady, 1991) that pulls all the participants together: nurses, physicians, interdisciplinary team members, patients, and family members. As a process structure of partnership between direct-care nurses and patients, shared governance provides a vehicle for improved communication, greater responsibility and accountability, and a way of coordinating, integrating, and facilitating care at the point of service that is relationship-based and patient-focused.

Patients respond positively when direct-care nurses partner with them in their care decisions. Some direct-care nurses make walking rounds during shift changes and intermittently throughout their shifts. They stop to speak with their patients each time and ask for their feedback, questions, concerns, and/or ideas. If the doctor came by earlier, they ask the patient what was said and listen to his or her report instead of telling the patient what the physician wrote in the chart or had told the nurse. These direct-care nurses invite patients who are able to do so to attend the interdisciplinary team meetings when the team members are discussing that patient's care. Engaging patients in conversation is one method of involving them in their own care. When direct-care nurses interact relationally with patients in partnership, patient and nurse satisfaction scores increase.

Nurses as partners in whole-systems shared governance

Nursing's role in whole-systems shared governance is multifaceted, occurring within multiple levels of the organization (i.e., macro-, meso-, and microsystems):

- Shared governance is a universal process structure or model. It can be applied in any setting. As it emerges in one division, it begins to affect other services, departments, and disciplines who want to participate in decisions that affect their future and roles, and want to be involved to the fullest extent possible as shared decision-making applies to them. That is be expected and anticipated.

- Other departments and disciplines should be implemented when they are ready. Although nurses generally lead the process change, shared governance will vary in terms of organizational application. When other departments are ready, nursing must be ready to assist, to encourage, and to act as role models, sharing the information and experiences gathered in their own implementation process. Allow the shared governance process model to materialize in the divisions, disciplines, and departments that seek it. (See Appendix 33: Interdisciplinary shared governance model.)

- Structure corporate and organizational integration into the shared governance process. Nursing support provides an opportunity for the organization to integrate everyone's growth in shared governance. Healthcare can only manage to change strategically if the whole organization joins nursing's efforts and they collectively undertake the necessary structures for change together. Shared governance needs to be incorporated so that it becomes an organizational imperative and continues to grow across the organization.

Many organizations have developed institutional process models (Porter-O'Grady, 1991), where all disciplines and departments have some role in making decisions that affect the direction and the operation of the organization. As individual disciplines do their work, they integrate with this larger process model (see Appendix 34: Shared governance work flow chart). All employees play a role in the organization as a whole, participating as part of the organization in the directions, policies, decisions, and objectives that set the organization on a course for its own future. Nursing has an opportunity to lead their respective organizations into that future through shared governance.

Shared governance process models and institutional models take on a number of different designs and are directed, in essence, to provide a framework so that members, divisions, and departments of the whole organization can participate together in seeking goals and objectives that guide their future. It is important that those organizations with such models emerge and begin to lead the future direction of the whole organization in providing a framework for integrative process models and shared decision-making.

Shared governance should be an integrating structure (Porter-O'Grady, 1991, 2004), then, that pulls all the participants together. It is a structure of partnership between manager and staff, between organization and discipline, between division and profession, and between worker and organization. It provides a vehicle for change, ownership, equity, investment, partnership, accountability, and for a way of coordinating, integrating, and facilitating the work of healthcare today and tomorrow.

A fundamental aspect of shared governance is the need to join all of the parties together in a venture to which they are all committed. The structural process and the emergent system is part of the design for a shared governance framework that will provide an integrative structure for collectively moving the organization toward desired outcomes. This is what needs to be done to lead strategic change.

The next step in the implementation of a shared governance process is to continue gathering information and resources to design, implement, and evaluate your own shared governance process. This book is designed to provide a broad base on which to build planning and implementation. Although there is no one "right" process model, the basic principles of shared governance are generic, viable, and measurable.

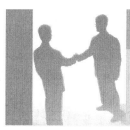

MEASURE YOUR PROCESS AND OUTCOMES AT THE POINT OF CARE

Contributing author: Robert Hess, PhD, RN, FAAN

Additional problems are the offspring of poor solutions.
— *Mark Twain*

Andrea, an emergency room nurse, felt overwhelmed. Her chief nursing officer had just promoted her to a newly created position of shared governance coordinator. She told Andrea to go forth and implement shared governance, which was expected to be a major component in the hospital's application for the American Nurses Credentialing Center (ANCC) Magnet Recognition Program® (MRP) status that was planned for next year. Andrea's anxiety stemmed from the fact that she had no idea what shared governance was, and none of the articles she had read explained the concept in a way that a real nurse could understand.

Shared governance's definition, assessment, and measurement have a history of vagueness, stretching from its initial conceptualization and implementation to subsequent evaluation. Anthony (2004) provides an overview of this complex organizational ambiguity. Dating from its roots—

when Luther Christman, PhD, RN, FAAN, spoke to the possibility of an autonomous nursing organization within a hospital at the 1975 American Nurses Association convention in Atlantic City, NJ—anecdotal accounts and research studies have attempted to connect shared governance with rosy outcomes. But without defining and measuring its underlying concept, governance, how can organizations assess how much of what is being shared, if at all? And if shared governance is not defined and measured, how can it be connected to outcomes?

Measurement Tools: Index of Professional Nursing Governance and Index of Professional Governance

Assessments and measurements of shared governance process models range from case study exemplars and implementation stories to research-based studies. Anthony (2004) provides an excellent overview of many of these studies. Anecdotal evidence of processes described in exemplars and case studies with subjective evaluations of outcomes provide a road map for designing and monitoring governance structures. Hess (1998) developed and validated an 86-item measurement instrument to evaluate the distribution of governance. He contended—then and now—that the extent of outcomes measurement determines if governance exists. Anything else is suspect.

Although Hess' tools have had limited use by other researchers, his Index of Professional Nursing Governance (IPNG, 1998) has been used to measure governance in healthcare organizations for more than 10 years (see Appendix 2). The IPNG evaluates the implementation of innovative management models and tracks changes in governance. The more global index, the Index of Professional Governance (IPG), measures the perceptions of all healthcare professionals within an organization (see Appendix 1).

The IPNG is the first and only quantitative measure of governance and its distribution among groups within healthcare organizations (Hess, 1998). This survey instrument uses 86 items to measure the balance of power, relying on a view of organizations as the rational and emergent systems described by the sociologist Alvin Gouldner (1959). In his classic analysis, Gouldner related the rational view of organizations as orderly formal structures with members who pursue the achievement of the acknowledged goals of the organization. This is the entity defined in organizational charts. However, an alternate organization, the emergent or natural organization, often exists outside of those charts. Natural structures emerge within an organization from groups with informal power that is hard to ignore. These groups sometimes pursue goals and agendas that are more relevant to them as professionals and not always aligned with the goals of the organization.

Specifically designed for nurses, the IPNG:

- Relies on the perceptions of the people surveyed within an organization to report not only which group has official authority over certain areas, but also which group has control and influence beyond the recognized and accepted order.

- Provides a baseline assessment of which groups have control and influence over vital organizational areas, such as professional practice and the resources that support it, before innovative organizational governance models are implemented. The survey tool can track changes in key areas during implementation, validate implementation, and provide benchmarks against other organizations.

- Compares governance scores of groups, such as management and staff and specific units or departments, within the organizations and provides guidance for those on the MRP journey.

- Offers the first opportunity to connect changes in governance to professional, clinical, and organizational outcomes across all micro- (unit-level), meso- (departments/divisions), and macrosystems (organizations).

The more global IPG is generic for all healthcare disciplines. During the last 17 years, both tools, the IPNG and the IPG, have been used in more than 100 hospitals, including several in the Middle Eastern countries of Lebanon and Jordan. The IPNG appears in more than 20 reported research studies. More than 20 MRP-status hospitals have used the IPNG to evaluate their progress in developing and/or establishing shared governance.

The IPNG is currently the most respected and frequently used measurement instrument for evaluating shared governance. For example, it is included in both ANCC's shared governance toolkit (Haag-Heitman & George, 2010) and the shared governance practice brief distributed to executives in member hospitals by the Advisory Board Company (2005), a think tank based in Washington, DC. The vast majority of these evaluations assess shared governance in single settings, using either cross-sectional or longitudinal time frames. Both IPNG and IPG instruments are reprinted in Appendixes 1 and 2 with permission. (See note at the end of this chapter on using these tools.)

Although no other instruments purport to measure governance across organizations, a few hospitals have created homegrown surveys to track implementation progress at their own institutions. For example, Havens created a valid and reliable governance-related instrument, the Decisional Involvement Scale, to measure actual and/or preferred decisional involvement of staff nurses and managers on nursing units, that has been used in several hospitals (Havens & Vasey, 2003).

Implementing a shared governance nursing practice model changes the organizational culture. Nursing shared governance moves any organization from a hierarchical structure in any form to a unit-level (unit-based), councilor, administrative, or congressional structural form that requires ongoing interdisciplinary collaboration, communication, flexibility, evaluation, and redesign of goals and processes.

The decision to assess the state of governance in an organization cannot be made lightly. Surveying staff brings up questions of confidentiality and can even be threatening to some, depending on the environment and how specific information can be to participants. For example, while unit-specific information can be important for strategic planning or targeted intervention, identifying units with just a few staff members can be viewed as compromising their anonymity. Some organizations may discover scores they had not anticipated, while others find their expectations validated.

Related literature and consultants alike are unclear about when and how often to assess or evaluate process or progress. Generally, the best time to assess governance is before implementation or revitalization of a program and again after a vital change has been affected. Most organizations measure change at about two-year intervals. One hospital assessed governance before implementation of a shared governance model and then annually thereafter. The administrators and staff put a lot of energy into their program. The scores validated the slow but steady progress of governance maturity. After a few years, survey scores demonstrated the organization placed firmly in the zone of shared governance.

Measuring governance with the IPNG before or during implementation can guide the creation of a strategic plan and refinement of the model. By tracking 86 individual items, participants can often identify those items with scores that can be improved on most easily and quickly within their particular organizational environments. Targeting items for change amounts to "teaching the test" because the items define governance. Changing them advances the resulting overall governance score.

 SHARED GOVERNANCE, SECOND EDITION

Research on the Evidence and Principles of Shared Governance

Destiny is not a matter of chance, it is a matter of choice; it is not a thing to be waited for,
it is a thing to be achieved.

— William Jennings Bryan

For those interested in learning more about the research and work done over the past 30 years on shared governance and leadership, there are some excellent articles and books available from the fields of business, management, economics, human resources, and healthcare. Anthony, Hess, Porter-O'Grady, Swihart, and others have studied the principles of shared governance and found them to be accurate delineators of nurse empowerment (Anthony, 2004; Howell et al., 2001; Porter-O'Grady, 2003a, 2003b, 2004, 2009a, 2009b, 2009c; Swihart, 2006). They and their colleagues have investigated multiple theoretical and empirical evidences to define shared governance and to determine whether or not a shared governance nursing practice model based on the principles of partnership, equity, accountability, and ownership achieves the positive outcomes desired.

Research on Shared Governance in a Government Agency

In a landmark study at the Durham VA Medical Center in North Carolina, Howell and his colleagues (2001) used the IPNG to study an established shared governance process model within a government agency, a highly bureaucratic and hierarchical organizational management system. They defined nursing governance as:

> *… multidimensional, encompassing the structure and process through which professional nurses in health care agencies control their professional practice and influence the organizational context in which it occurs … [and] loosely described shared governance as a system of structuring nursing practice that gives nurses at the bedside the responsibility for decision related to their practice. In the words of Prater, it implies the allocation of control, power, or authority (governance) among mutually (shared) interested and vested parties. (pp. 187–188)*

Six dimensions for measurement

The researchers studied 183 RNs in nursing service at the Durham VA Medical Center (273 surveys were distributed but only 183 returned). They used Hess' 86-item instrument IPNG to measure nurses' perceptions of professional nursing governance facilitywide on a continuum ranging from traditional (dominant group is nursing management/administration) to shared (decision-making shared between direct-care nurses and management/administration) to look at the following six dimensions with subscales:

1. **Nursing personnel:** Who controls nursing personnel by hiring, promoting, evaluating, recommending, adjusting salaries and benefits, formulating unit budgets, creating new positions, conducting disciplinary action, and making terminations

2. **Information:** Who has access to information relevant to governance activities, such as opinions of managers, staff nurses, physicians, patients, and interdisciplinary team members; unit budgets and expenditures; nursing service goals and objectives; and the organization's finances, compliance reports, and strategic plan

3. **Goals:** Who sets goals and negotiates the resolution of conflict at different organizational levels among nurses, other members of the interdisciplinary healthcare team, and organizational leadership, as well as philosophy, goals, objectives, and a formal grievance procedure

4. **Resources:** Who influences the resources that support professional practice: monitoring and securing supplies, recommending and consulting other services, determining daily assignments, and regulating patient movements (admissions, transfers, referrals, placements, and discharges)

5. **Participation:** Who creates and participates in committee structures related to governance activities, such as committees that address policies and procedures for clinical practice, staffing, scheduling, budgeting, and collaboration

6. **Practice:** Who controls professional practice in terms of patient care standards, standards of professional practice and care, quality, staffing levels, qualifications, competency, professional development and education requirements, and evidence-based practice (incorporating research into practice)

Higher scores on any of these six subscales indicated that staff nurses perceived themselves to have greater influence over professional decision-making in their organization. Scores for three of the six dimensions (nursing personnel, information, and goals) were consistent with a traditional governance environment, although the scores on information and goals were very close to the shared governance range. In the other three dimensions (participation, resources, and practice), nurses perceived a significant shift toward shared governance with scores near or higher than the base range for shared governance.

The results of this study demonstrated that "shared governance within several critical areas of nursing practice can be successfully implemented" within an organizational structure thought to be traditional and bureaucratic (Howell et al., 2001, p. 195). This study demonstrates that shared governance can be implemented in any organization or practice setting, although the degree to which it is implemented and its characteristics may be shaped by each unique environment. Shared governance can and will look different in every organization.

Further research using valid instruments such as the IPNG must examine outcomes associated with varying levels of implementation of shared governance and its role in the recruitment and retention of nurses. As medical care is integrated into healthcare systems, community-based outpatient centers, and cybertechnologies that triage and treat patients across cyberspace, staff nurses are becoming more involved in shared decision-making. What impact will shared governance have on the professional practice environment of care for new generations of nurses in a sociotechnological era? The IPG is now being used to assess physicians' and allied health disciplines' involvement in shared governance in hospitals, as well as commercial entities involved in healthcare. Its use in determining patient involvement is not far off.

Research on measuring shared governance

Following are a few more references related to the research, development, and/or use of the IPNG for those interested in exploring this work further, accessed online March 19, 2011, at *www.sharedgovernance.org/ipngarticles.htm* from the Forum for Shared Governance (*www.sharedgovernance.org*): Anderson (2000); Barden (2009); Brooks et al. (2005); George, Burke, & Rodgers (1997); Haag-Heitman & George (2010); Hess (1994a, 1994b, 1996a, 1996b, 1998a, 1998b, 2004); Howell et al. (2001); Kang (1995); Lee (1998); Lee, Yang, Lee, & Wu (2001); Lee, Yang, Wu, & Lee (2001); Nursing Executive Center Practice Brief (2005); Pettitt (2002); Singh (2010); Staff (1996); Swihart (2006); Weston (2006).

See the expanded bibliography for many additional resources and references related to seminal and current research done on shared governance structure, processes, and outcomes.

Note on using the IPNG and IPG

The subscales keys, which are necessary to interpret the IPNG and the IPG, are proprietary but available for a nominal charge to researchers, clinicians, and administrators who formally request permission and agree to adhere to guidelines for use. Free use of the instrument may be available for graduate students and researchers, particularly those conducting outcomes investigations. Revenue generated from the use of the IPNG and IPG is used to support the work of the Forum for Shared Governance and the development and maintenance of its website, *www.sharedgovernance.org.*

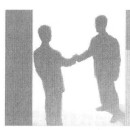

CASE STUDIES: SNAPSHOTS OF SHARED GOVERNANCE AND BEST PRACTICES

After reading this chapter, the participant should be able to:

- Describe the attributes of the shared governance processes of the organizations featured in the case studies

Implementing Shared Governance in U.S. and Global Communities

Shared governance takes on different shapes in various organizations because of the unique culture of each institution. However, if organizations remain true to the principles in their design, implementation, and evolution, then they share the basic elements, or attributes, of shared governance—they are just rolled out in different ways. For example, this chapter details the inner workings of shared governance in three vastly different hospitals. Consider how the process is similar despite the difference in size and setting.

Case Study 1: Saint Joseph's Hospital, Atlanta

Background

Saint Joseph's Hospital (SJH) in Atlanta is a 410-bed tertiary care hospital. In the late 1970s and early '80s, due to the repercussions of relocation and increased competition, SJH's nursing vacancy rate hovered at nearly 20% and turnover around 35%. Patient satisfaction was low, and quality was problematic in some areas. We needed a fresh start.

SJH's journey toward developing a distinguished nursing organization began when the nursing division implemented shared governance as the professional practice model (PPM). The decision to implement shared governance resulted from a commitment to make SJH a place where nurses could work with significant autonomy.

Implementation

Knowing that nurses desired control over practices and procedures that affected direct care, we identified several priority areas in our search for a structure, including education, quality assurance, management, and standards for practice. These four areas served as the basis for our original shared governance councils.

Education council

Responsible for professional development:

+ Arranged educational programming for the units

+ Developed educational programs for practice changes

+ Created patient education materials

Quality assurance council

Responsible for comparing nursing practice to current standards and determining the rate of compliance:

+ Coordinated ongoing compliance measurement activities

+ Made suggestions to standards about deficits in practice

Management council

Nursing leadership is responsible for securing material, fiscal, and human resources and for enforcing compliance with work developed by the three staff councils:

+ Secured adequate staffing and determined staffing matrices based on patient needs

+ Budgeted for nursing care

Nursing standards council

Responsible for nursing process assessment, plan, intervention, and evaluation:

+ Developed standards, policies, and procedures that govern nursing care

+ Developed the care delivery model

Best practices to handle the nitty-gritty

Determining council membership

The council model was developed by a team of staff and nursing leadership. Once the council structure was determined, membership criteria needed to be developed and members selected. Prospective members for the staff councils completed applications for membership (just as we do today) and were selected by the development team. Currently, members are selected for a two-year term and rotate in either October or April, thus limiting the amount of turnover at one time. The chair and vice chair each serve for two years, so the longest possible term one can serve on a council is six years. Once the nursing division council model was assigned and implemented, each nursing unit was expected to develop a similar structure.

When they were formed, the councils had eight to 12 members. As the model matured, these members were often forwarded for membership by their respective unit-based governance committees. On the staff councils, only the staff RNs could vote with a leader serving as an advisor. Clinical nurse specialists were also assigned to a council for support, without voting privileges. Also, the councils asked other hospital professionals to serve in advisory, nonvoting capacities (e.g., the hospital quality assurance/performance improvement coordinator serves as an advisor to the nursing quality assurance council). Councils also invited other hospital staff to attend council meetings, as needed (e.g., nursing informatics staff are invited to standards council meetings to determine online charting practices).

Ensuring staff involvement in council activities

Council members represented several areas to control the size of councils and to enhance the council's ability to develop an effective team. Initially, motivation among peers and replacement of RNs who spent time off the unit to participate in council activities fueled involvement in shared governance. At the time, the usual workday was eight hours, so a staff council member was paid eight hours to participate in council day. The council meetings usually lasted about six hours, with the other two hours for council work completed outside the council meeting.

Due to the significant commitment required of the council chair, the council chair was paid for two eight-hour days each month and was also freed from clinical responsibilities during these times. The chair's manager must ensure that he or she is relieved of bedside responsibilities during the council meeting.

In 1985, the standards council developed and implemented a clinical ladder/levels advancement process. In developing the ladder, this council awarded points for various activities that support shared governance. Council membership grew so popular that the bylaws had to specify that a period of six months had to elapse before applying for membership on another staff council.

Developing leadership skills

Ensuring competency among council leadership was then and remains today the greatest challenge to the shared governance model. To address leadership competency and at the request of staff nurses, the vice chair position was developed to help inculcate understanding of the necessary leadership abilities of council chairs. Various programs were developed to help with leadership development (e.g., leadership classes, team leading). Each council also has a leadership advisor who does not vote but who is present for leadership mentoring.

Closing the communication loop

A year after all of the councils started, it became clear that there was a lack of communication between councils, especially as there were no shared members (e.g., no staff member could be a member of more than one council at a time). This difficulty in "closing the loop" led to the creation of the coordinating council. This council is made up of the chairs of each shared governance council and a handful of other nurse leaders. A staff nurse elected by peers chairs this committee. The coordinating council was responsible for coordinating council activities, setting the nursing strategic plan, developing and revising the nursing staff bylaws for annual staff vote, and preparing the staff to select the guiding nursing theory for nursing services.

An evolving process

Note: The following is partially adapted from Sharkey, K. (2005). "Embody nursing excellence through change: Why a designated hospital aligned its PPM with the 14 Forces." **HCPro's Advisor** *to the ANCC Magnet Recognition Program® 1(8): 7–8.*

Until 2004, there were relatively few changes made to the initial council structure, which included changing council names (see Figure 7.1), modifying supporting councils, and increasing council responsibilities.

When SJH first developed its shared governance model, it created a nursing research forum as a subcommittee of the nursing performance improvement council. Nurses of all educational levels who supported nursing research within the facility served on this subcommittee. Although this structure was effective at the time, SJH recognized the need to assess our PPM's infrastructure continuously to keep it energized and focused in the face of emerging challenges.

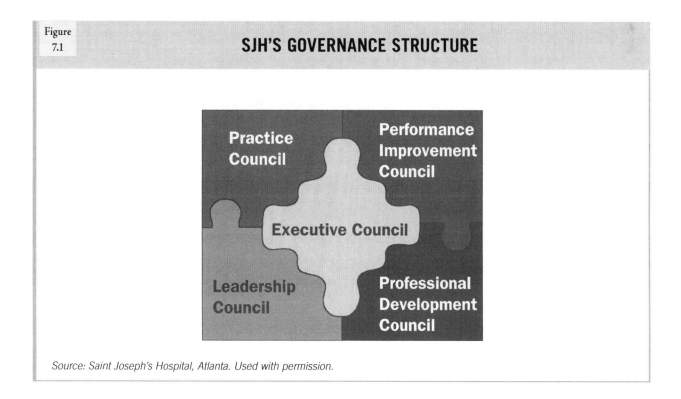

Figure 7.1

SJH'S GOVERNANCE STRUCTURE

Practice Council

Performance Improvement Council

Executive Council

Leadership Council

Professional Development Council

Source: Saint Joseph's Hospital, Atlanta. Used with permission.

Therefore, in 2004, the nursing division aligned its own strategic plan with the organization's strategic plan to focus on completing both nursing and hospitalwide goals. Several of the strategic initiatives developed for nursing focused on research projects and, because SJH is an American Nurses Credentialing Center (ANCC) Magnet Recognition Program® (MRP)–designated organization, increasing staff awareness of how the Forces of Magnetism applied in their daily practice. For the first time in 25 years, SJH made a significant change within its PPM by eliminating the nursing research forum and expanding the PPM to include a sixth independent council devoted to nursing research.

Last year, the executive council, which sits at the core of the PPM, made the motion to change the bylaws to create that sixth council. The staff nurses voted to accept this change. SJH redesigned the conceptual model of shared governance to portray the relationship that the research council would have with all the other councils. To complete the process, each council was aligned with the Forces that it best represents. This new model is the focal point of discussion during nursing orientation because it clearly depicts the interrelation between our PPM and the tenets of the MRP (see Figure 7.2).

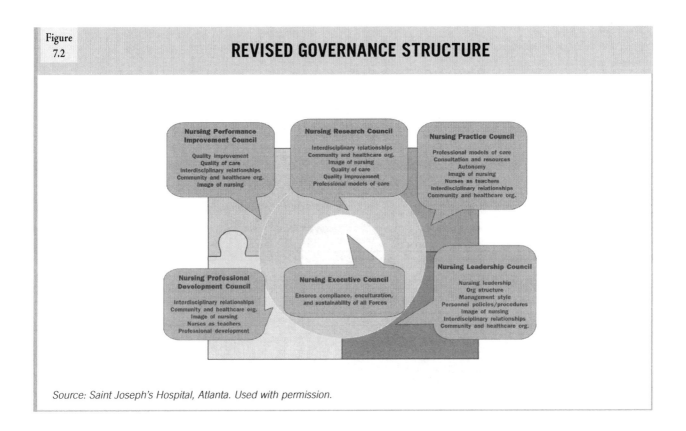

Figure 7.2

REVISED GOVERNANCE STRUCTURE

Source: Saint Joseph's Hospital, Atlanta. Used with permission.

    SHARED GOVERNANCE, SECOND EDITION

In 2005, we celebrated our 25th anniversary of shared governance. Members of the nursing staff have remained vigilant over the years to ensure that our model holds true to the concept of shared decision-making. Decisions about direct care must remain in the hands of those who provide it, although it is not always easy to discern where responsibility for all types of decisions lies.

Looking back over the years, we are struck by the elegance of SJH's shared governance process model, which was implemented by Sharon Finnigan and Tim Porter-O'Grady when they were newly appointed nurse leaders at SJH. Their energy and enthusiasm not only generated interest and restored a sense of pride to much of our nursing staff at the time of implementation, but it also inspired us to ensure that shared governance flourishes in our nursing environment over time, and throughout change.

Case Study 2: Southwestern Vermont Medical Center, Bennington

Background

As part of its journey to elevate the professional role and recognition of the RN, Southwestern Vermont Medical Center (SVMC)—a 99-bed community hospital in rural Vermont—undertook an ambitious campaign to decentralize the nursing department and empower the direct-care RN. One step in that process was the development and implementation of a shared governance model of professional practice.

In 1994, SVMC formed a shared governance steering committee, consisting of RNs from each nursing unit, two nursing directors, and the chief nurse executive. The steering committee explored models of shared decision-making and became interested in Tim Porter-O'Grady's councilor model of shared governance. Convinced that this model would support the goals established by the steering committee, Porter-O'Grady was invited to present his model to the nursing staff at SVMC. More than 60 nurses attended the program, and it gave the staff the vision and energy they needed to move forward with the development of their shared governance model.

Implementation

The shared governance model that was implemented in 1994 mirrored the Porter-O'Grady model, as described in his book, *Implementing Shared Governance: Creating a Professional Organization* (1992). It consisted of four primary councils—practice, management, education, and quality—and a coordinating council, which facilitated the communication between the other four councils.

Membership within the practice, education, and quality councils included staff nurses from each of the nursing units and a nursing director. A staff nurse chaired each council. The management council included all of the nursing directors, the chief nursing officer (CNO), four staff nurses, and a nursing director who served as the chair. The coordinating council's membership included the chairs of each council in addition to the CNO, who served as chair.

Original structure and responsibilities

The original roles and responsibilities of each of the councils are described in the following sections.

Practice council

Role: The professional practice council defines the parameters of clinical practice. It is the primary decision-making body related to clinical issues within a professional framework.

Responsibilities: The function of the professional practice council includes but is not limited to the following:

- Standards of care and practice: To oversee the development, implementation, review, revision, and approval of standards of care and practice at SVMC, including, but not limited to, procedures, protocols, and guidelines

- Clinical advancement: To oversee the clinical advancement program and provide direction for structure, finance, and the appeals process

- Peer review: To review the process of evaluating professional accountability, including, but not limited to, peer review, job descriptions, and performance appraisals

- Delivery of care: To provide direction for delivery of care

- Resource utilization: To make recommendations for resource utilization (e.g., staffing, budget, product selection, capital purchases, and professional development)

- Information systems: To collaborate with nursing information systems on issues that interface with nursing practice

Management council

Role: The management council supports, facilitates, and integrates the mission, vision, and values of Southwestern Vermont Health Care (SVHC), our corporate organization, with the philosophy of professional nursing practice.

Responsibilities: The function of the management council includes but is not limited to the following:

- Development, implementation, review, and revision of nursing department policies

- Establishment and maintenance of practices that ensure fiscal viability in a managed care environment

+ Development and implementation of cost accounting systems to achieve cost reductions

+ Identification of staff learning needs to facilitate practice in a managed care environment

+ Establishment and maintenance of staffing patterns to meet the needs of defined patient populations

+ Integration of Joint Commission and other regulatory agency standards into practice

+ Oversight of the development and implementation of patient care standards

+ Appointment of nursing representative(s) to the employee participation committee

+ Participation in the development of the SVMC strategic plan

+ Establishment of annual nursing department goals to achieve the SVHC strategic plan, the hospital's annual operational objectives, and the continued development of professional practice

+ Support of the SVHC/SVMC mission, vision, and values through program and service development

Education council

Role: The education council provides direction for nursing education to promote optimal professional competencies.

Responsibilities: The function of the education council includes but is not limited to the following:

+ Identify long- and short-term educational goals

+ Facilitate education related to quality issues and practice issues

+ Facilitate communication related to new products, pharmaceuticals, and new policies

+ Facilitate communication of unit-based educational programming and competencies

+ Maintain communication with the multidisciplinary education committee

+ Meet with nursing educators who use the hospital as a clinical site at least annually to influence curricula and to improve learning experiences

Quality council

Role: The quality council oversees and coordinates nursing performance improvement/continuous quality improvement activities to support the SVMC mission, vision, values, and annual performance improvement plan using an interdisciplinary approach.

Responsibilities: The function of the quality council includes but is not limited to the following:

- Establish monitors for identified patient care and nursing practice standards to ensure compliance

- Evaluate monitors that continue out of compliance for more than one quarter

- Act as a resource and provide education for unit-based quality improvement functions

- Perform root cause analysis for all nursing sentinel events

Refining the vision

In 1997, three years after the shared governance model was implemented at SVMC, the first major modifications to the program occurred. At the coordinating council's annual review of the professional practice bylaws, which define the shared governance model, staff discussed their feelings of a disconnect between the management and practice councils. Nursing procedures were developed, reviewed, and revised at practice council, but the supporting policy was the responsibility of management council.

Staff also expressed a desire to have a stronger voice in areas that governed the professional work environment, such as scheduling, staffing patterns, and vacation time. At this meeting, a decision was made to merge management and practice councils into one and to name this new group the leadership council. The membership for this council included a staff nurse representative from each nursing unit, all nursing directors, and clinical nurse specialists.

An interdisciplinary shift

In 1999, the second major change in the shared governance model began. The need for greater interdisciplinary collaboration in clinical practice was becoming apparent. To support the goal of having all clinical departments work together to drive best patient outcomes, it was decided to move to an interdisciplinary model of shared decision-making. The CNO was also the chief operating officer, with responsibility for all clinical departments, which facilitated this move. The revision of the shared governance model into an interdisciplinary model was recognized as a significant change, requiring buy-in from the other clinical areas as well as from nursing. The transition of the councils was set to occur over a one-year period, with one council at a time moving to the interdisciplinary structure.

New structure and responsibilities

The process was completed in early 2002, taking a little more time than anticipated. The new council structure and responsibilities are described in the following sections.

Leadership council

Role: The leadership council supports, facilitates, and integrates the mission, vision, and values of SVHC with the philosophy of professional nursing practice.

It defines the parameters for clinical practice and is the primary decision-making body related to management and clinical practice.

Responsibilities: The function of the leadership council includes but is not limited to the following:

+ Develop, implement, review, and revise nursing department policies, procedures, standards of care, guidelines, and protocols to meet Joint Commission and other regulatory guidelines.

+ Establish and maintain systems that ensure fiscal viability.

+ Provide input and leadership in the development of the strategic plan.

+ Provide direction for clinical advancement and peer review process.

+ Provide leadership and direction for evaluation and modification of the care delivery system.

+ Provide direction and guidance for the selection and implementation of nursing information systems.

+ Work collaboratively with the department of human resources on recruitment and retention activities.

+ Appoint nursing representative(s) to employee participation committee.

+ Establish annual nursing department goals to achieve the SVHC strategic plan, the SVMC's annual operational objectives, and the continued development of professional practice.

- Ensure that nursing procedures are developed, reviewed, and revised in an evidence-based process, using current research, standards of care, and best practice findings. Existing procedures are reviewed and revised as necessary every three years, or more often as needed, per Joint Commission standards:

  – The procedure review committee is operationally accountable to the leadership council. The procedure review committee, through leadership council, has access to the resources needed to ensure that the most current evidence and literature are available for review.

  – Membership of the procedure review committee includes representation from each nursing unit. The committee is chaired by a clinical nurse specialist and meets at least quarterly.

  – Specialty-specific procedures are developed, reviewed, and revised at the unit level. Appropriate resources to support the evidence-based approach are available through the unit-based budgets.

Clinical education council

Role: The clinical education council serves as the mechanism for defining educational needs throughout the hospital. As needs are defined, the education council will ensure that individuals/departments create programs/plans to meet the identified needs.

The council is responsible to the director of education for ensuring compliance with regulatory requirements and other education-related mandates.

Responsibilities are as follows:

- Establish educational priorities based on regulatory requirements and identified learning needs

- Ensure compliance with mandatory educational programming

- Oversee implementation of departmental education plans

Clinical quality

Role and responsibilities: The clinical quality council oversees and coordinates nursing and other clinical performance improvement activities to support the hospital's mission, vision, and values and to uphold the functions of the hospital's performance improvement plan using an interdisciplinary approach. As such, the council does the following:

◆ Establishes, reviews, and/or helps to revise monitors for identified patient care and nursing practice standards to ensure compliance

◆ Evaluates monitors that are out of compliance or below threshold for more than one quarter to ensure that there is an adequate corrective action plan to make and sustain improvement

◆ Acts as a resource to provide education for unit-based and departmental quality improvement functions

◆ Evaluates trends and coordinates efforts to make recommended improvements

◆ Reports on trends, findings, improvement opportunities, and accomplishments through representation on the hospital's performance improvement committee

Coordinating council

Role: The coordinating council ensures the overall coordination of the activities of the other councils and is accountable for the integration of services and decisions that affect the nursing department and other clinical departments. The coordinating council will integrate the SVHC mission, vision, and strategic goals into the nursing department plan.

Responsibilities: The function of the coordinating council includes but is not limited to the following:

◆ Review monthly minutes from all councils

◆ Ensure two-way communication to all councils, staff, and administration

◆ Problem-solve issues referred by councils

◆ Review professional practice bylaws and nursing department plan of care annually

◆ Support the development and implementation of unit-based councils

◆ Monitor ongoing progress toward achievement of department goals

Shared governance in action

The interdisciplinary focus of the PPM of shared decision-making has improved communication and collaboration among all disciplines. Physician leadership recognizes the leadership council as the decision-making body for the clinical departments and uses this council to develop patient care protocols, medical staff policies, and physician orders. For example, when the pharmacy and therapeutics committee (which is a medical staff committee) decided to develop a glycemic control protocol, it used the leadership council for input into nursing and pharmacy's responsibility within the protocol. This collaboration allowed for the creation of a protocol that respects the roles and responsibilities of each clinical department.

As another example, the chair of clinical quality reported on the lack of progress by individual nursing units to reduce medication errors at the coordinating council. Recognizing that it needed to address medication errors from a broader perspective, the coordinating council established a medication error task force, which included staff nurses, a nursing director, and the director of pharmacy. This group conducted an in-depth analysis of medication errors and reported back to leadership council with recommendations on system changes to improve the safe administration of medications.

An evolving process

The shared governance model of professional practice at SVMC has continued to evolve and mature. Each nursing department has developed its unique unit-based model that supports the larger model. All nursing units and most of the other clinical departments have self-scheduling models in place. Staff nurses are responsible for the shift-to-shift adjustments in staffing based on their professional knowledge and judgment as to the care needs of patients. An example of how one unit has continued to evolve its shared governance model is the peer support team (PST) developed by SVMC's women's and children's unit. The purpose of the PST is to resolve issues or conflicts that arise between staff regarding professional behavior/conduct before the matters require intervention from the department director. The PST consists of three staff nurses—one from each shift—who are selected by their peers. Educated on conflict management and negotiation, the team approaches each case referred to them with the intention of resolving the issue so staff feel supported and respected. Nursing directors support the SVMC shared governance model, as it allows them to focus on broader organizational strategic initiatives. Nurses and other clinicians express satisfaction with their ability to voice concerns, put forth new ideas, and participate in decisions that affect both their clinical practice and the professional work environment.

Case Study 3: King Hussein Cancer Center, Amman, Jordan

Contributor: Majeda Afeef, PhD(c), MSN, RN, director of nursing services, King Hussein Cancer Center, Amman, Jordan

This example details the inner workings of shared governance in the King Hussein Cancer Center (KHCC) in Amman, Jordan. Consider how the process is similar as it unfolds despite the differences in culture and practice setting.

Background

KHCC was founded in 1997 as Al-Amal Cancer Center, which means "the center of hope" in Arabic. In 2002, there was an official ceremony to change the name of the center to honor the late King Hussein, who had died of cancer.

KHCC became one of the leading regional medical facilities in the Middle East providing comprehensive cancer care to both adult and pediatric patients. It is a 170-bed center that delivers the latest in cancer treatment to patients, actively promoting awareness and educational programs for early detection and prevention of cancer as well as training and research to decrease mortality and alleviate the suffering that results from cancer.

Nursing services began with the establishment of KHCC in 2002. The focus then was on building nursing manpower and maximizing the capabilities of nurses by training and mentorship. Preparation for the Joint Commission International Accreditation (JCIA) process began at that time, too, to ensure delivery of the highest quality of care in a safe environment. In 2006, the center was the first institution in Jordan accredited by JCIA. Nurses at KHCC emphasized quality assurance activities and enforced a culture of safety and quality for patient care. In 2009, the nurses started their formal journey toward MRP excellence by implementing shared governance, establishing nursing research, and promoting evidence-based nursing practice at the unit level. The decision to implement shared governance resulted from a commitment to make KHCC a place where nurses could practice with autonomy to achieve the best outcomes relative to patient care and the profession of nursing.

Evolution of shared governance management process

Early steps started in understanding the concept and evolving the processes of shared governance by spreading the word among nursing leadership and direct-care nurses. We increased their education and awareness by providing them resources and opportunities to talk about this new paradigm. Nursing leadership and the MRP project coordinator attended the annual ANCC MRP conferences, which helped to increase awareness and build relationships with different institutions who also implemented shared governance. Meeting with the founder of the Forum for Shared Governance, Dr. Robert Hess, during one of the MRP conferences helped in better understanding shared governance and how his tool, the Index of Professional Nursing Governance (IPNG), works to measure the development of shared governance in the organization.

KHCC nurses' perceptions about shared governance was assessed using the IPNG before implementing any structure of shared governance in nursing as a baseline and will be assessed repeatedly throughout the journey. Nursing's total score for the first IPNG was 181.64 (range for shared governance is 173 to 344), showing that decision-making is a shared process between direct-care nurses and managers. However, the breakdown into the six domains indicated that nurses perceived that although they are sharing in some decisions with the nursing management team, the reason was their involvement in accreditation processes and quality assurance initiatives in nursing services rather than decisions related to their professional practice, quality, and competence.

Introduction of shared governance in unit-level leadership

As the awareness was increased among the nursing team regarding shared governance, it was introduced gradually in different patient care units by establishing unit-level councils. These councils are chaired by direct-care nurses who are coached by their unit managers and encouraged to facilitate their council meetings. This allows better understanding and involvement from nurses at all levels. Additionally, all chairs attend a comprehensive workshop about handling unit meetings and team communication. Other nurses in the unit are encouraged to communicate their questions, concerns, and/or issues with the chair as part of an outline for the meeting agenda.

In the early stages of building the unit-level councils, the focus of discussion was unit operations with little focus on issues regarding patient care. However, nurses were encouraged to keep meeting and were helped and supported by nursing leadership to have group work with all unit-level council chairs to draft an initial and basic framework with responsibilities for the unit councils, which was successfully and enthusiastically accomplished (see Figure 7.3).

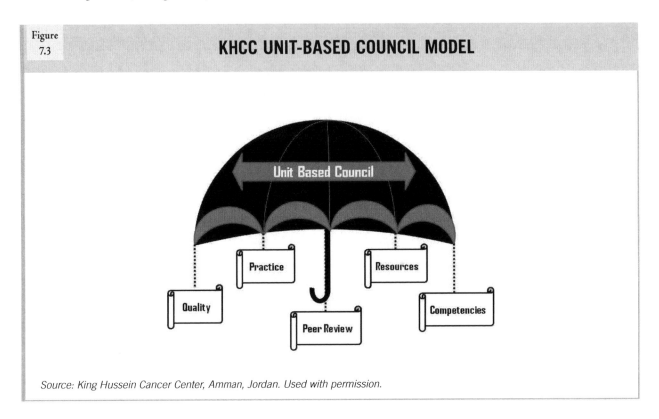

Figure 7.3

KHCC UNIT-BASED COUNCIL MODEL

Source: King Hussein Cancer Center, Amman, Jordan. Used with permission.

The unit-level council is responsible for:

+ Encouraging communication, collaboration, innovation, and collegiality in all patient care issues and working environments in the unit

+ Facilitating the continuous development and improvement in quality of care provided, competencies of the nurses, and excellence of practice in the unit

+ Supporting and encouraging mentorships for nurses at all levels

Building awareness about shared governance was continued throughout the process. For example, an international consultant was invited to give more education about shared governance and transformational leadership and to evaluate the work that had been done in the unit-level councils. Resources have been allocated by the general director, the director of nurses, and many supporters throughout KHCC, including library services, nursing education, human resources, and others.

Implementation

After establishment of a unit council charter and framework, the need for a bigger "umbrella" to oversee and coordinate all activities of the unit councils was identified. Taking input of direct-care nurses to a higher level of responsibility and execution or coordination evolved. By the end of 2010, the taskforce team (design team/steering committee) had established six governing councils and a coordinating council structure (see Figure 7.4). All governing councils are chaired by a nurse manager and cochaired by a direct-care nurse for the first six months to mentor them into their new roles, responsibilities, and accountabilities related to shared governance. Then, the leadership of the council will be passed to the direct-care nurses. This approach was adopted to ensure enough time to mentor the direct-care nurses and to alleviate some of the anxiety they expressed from being given these new roles.

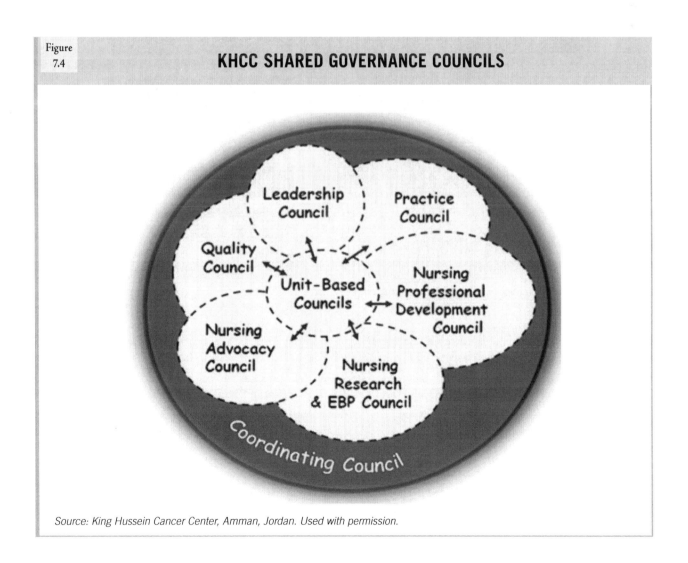

Figure 7.4

KHCC SHARED GOVERNANCE COUNCILS

Source: King Hussein Cancer Center, Amman, Jordan. Used with permission.

Unlike many western countries, many nurses in Jordan are younger in age with less experience in nursing practice. At KHCC, the average age for the nurses is 25 years old with three years of nursing practice experience after graduation from nursing school.

Shared governance was integrated into the PPM, which was developed by a taskforce team of direct-care nurses and nurse managers in 2010 and involved integration of system theory and campus theory (see Figure 7.5).

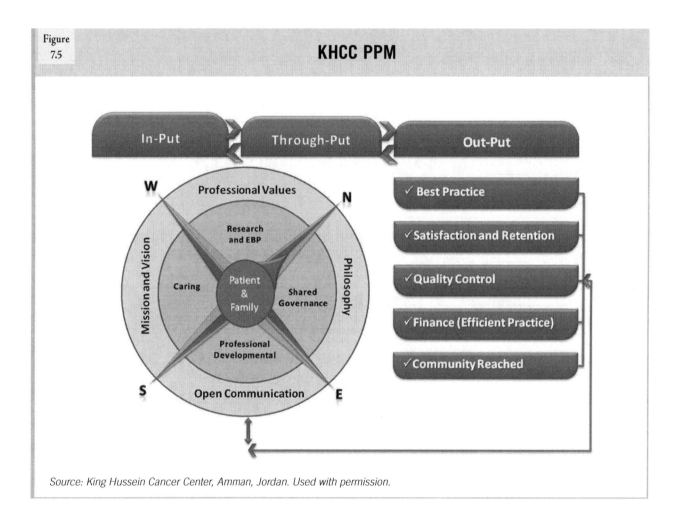

Figure 7.5

KHCC PPM

Source: King Hussein Cancer Center, Amman, Jordan. Used with permission.

Professional development council

This council is responsible for professional development, including the following:

+ Determine educational needs for all nursing staff at all levels; categories include new nursing orientees, preceptors, and staff orientation

- Facilitate direct-care nurse development

- Develop a nursing service newsletter

- Assess clinical education needs of nurses at all levels and develop strategies to meet those needs in collaboration with the nursing practice council, as well as education and training center

- Participate in the development of competency-based orientation programs, including the annual competency review process, in conjunction with the clinical practice council and unit-level councils

- Facilitate and enhance the process of nurses' certifications

- Assess and evaluate the professional practice model of nursing at KHCC and participate in the development of educational programs to assist nursing staff in the implementation of the nursing care delivery system

- Identify priorities and make recommendations related to leadership development programs

- Foster an environment conducive to the advancement and utilization of nursing research in collaboration with the nursing research and evidence-based practice (EBP) council

- Assess and evaluate the effectiveness of the professional nurse advancement ladder

Nursing quality and performance improvement council

This council is responsible for quality of nursing care and performance improvement:

- Coordinate the performance improvement and patient safety activities as delegated by the KHCC quality council, with particular emphasis on systems improvements related to nursing practices and care outcomes

- Develop, revise, and approve the annual nursing quality improvement plan, along with completing an annual evaluation of the effectiveness of the plan

- Endorse and monitor department and unit-level quality improvement plans

- Integrate the nursing quality improvement process with the hospital plan to detect trends and patterns of performance that affect more than one department or service

- Review and evaluate data (National Database of Nursing Quality Indicators, unit audit data, benchmarks) and use the data to develop action plans in collaboration with unit practice councils in the department of nursing to ensure quality patient outcomes

- Collaborate with other disciplines to monitor and evaluate compliance to standards and make recommendations to enhance continuous quality improvement and safety

- Monitor and analyze data relative to nursing quality and safety practices seeking opportunities for continual improvement; evaluate outcomes in conjunction with these initiatives

- Monitor the appropriateness and effectiveness of the care provided by the nursing staff while assessing and ensuring compliance with established standards of care and practice

- Monitor RN satisfaction by adapting the tool, conducting periodic surveys, and analyzing and benchmarking outcomes

Nursing practice council

This council is responsible for maintaining the following standards of clinical nursing practice:

- Provide input for the revision and approval of nursing documentation standards

- Consult on the redesign of the hospital patient care delivery systems

- Review, revise, and approve policies, procedures, and standards of care; incorporate nursing research findings into clinical practice in collaboration with the nursing research and EBP council

- Consult and collaborate on interdisciplinary issues that impact patient care

- Participate in reviews and communication regarding new clinical products and equipment

- Implement peer-review strategies

- Integrate professional practice model dimensions into all aspects of nursing practice

Nursing research and EBP council

This council is responsible for integrating nursing research and EBP into clinical and operational processes at point of care:

- Provide a nursing forum for creative and innovative thinking in collaboration with nursing committees, councils, and staff members for identifying, initiating, conducting, and publishing nursing research and EBP projects

- Enable nurses at all levels to appropriately explore the safest and best practices for their patients and practice environments and to generate new knowledge

- Assist nurses at all levels in evaluating and using published research findings in their practice and at point of care

- Ensure that knowledge gained through nursing research and EBP is disseminated to nurses at all levels

- Assist nurses with the preparation of research proposals and Institutional Review Board applications

- Participate in educating the nurses at all levels

- Create guidelines to enhance EBP understanding (journal clubs, group discussions)

- Mentor nurses at all levels to explore, evaluate, conduct, and publish nursing research

- Facilitate research partnerships with colleges/universities

Nursing advocacy council

This council is responsible for organizing and maintaining the recognition, recruitment, advancement, rewards, clinical ladder, rewards, and recruitment of nurses:

- Promote the recruitment and retention of professional nurses and support staff within KHCC

- Create nursing recognitions in collaboration with the professional development council

- Support the elements for empowering a professional nursing practice environment

- Review and update the career development ladder

+ Identify innovative staff recognition and reward strategies

+ Maintain and strengthen the relationship with other disciplines

Coordinating council

This council is responsible for provision of leadership and direction to all nursing councils:

+ Ensure nursing representation on hospital interdisciplinary decision-making committees and councils

+ Delegate initiatives to the appropriate nursing council(s)

+ Review and approve recommended revisions to all nursing council bylaws

+ Provide guidance and support to the chairs and chair-elects of all nursing governance councils

+ Review the annual report submitted by each nursing council and provide feedback and direction based on information submitted

+ Oversee the shared governance process to ensure maximum efficiency and effectiveness

+ Develop a strategic plan for nursing across the KHCC

+ Develop and periodically revise nursing strategic vision and philosophy statements

+ Support shared governance among nursing staff

+ Communicate and follow-up all other councils' activities with the higher decision-making councils and/or committees if required

+ Assign placement of new councils, committees, or groups within the shared governance structure

Although KHCC nurses still need much emphasis on awareness and training regarding shared governance and transformational leadership, they show an eager acceptance of the required changes and a ready willingness to learn. Although they are already exceptional nurses, they want to be even better, the best nurses possible, and are proud of the services they give to all their patients and families. They believe shared governance will help them achieve their goals through collaborative professional relationships with their interprofessional and interdisciplinary team members, patients and families, and ever-widening global communities of practice.

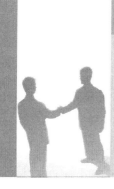

RELATIONSHIPS FOR EXCELLENCE: ANCC MAGNET RECOGNITION PROGRAM® AND INTERNATIONAL ORGANIZATION FOR STANDARDIZATION 9001: 2008 QUALITY MANAGEMENT

LEARNING OBJECTIVES

After reading this chapter, the participant should be able to:

- Describe the American Nurses Credentialing Center Magnet Recognition Program® and its relationship to shared governance

- Describe the International Organization for Standardization 9001:2008 quality management system and its relationship to shared governance

I find the important thing in life is not where we are, but in what direction we are moving.

– Oliver Wendell Holmes

The Relationship Between Shared Governance and the ANCC Magnet Recognition Program®

The mission of the American Nurses Credentialing Center (ANCC) is to promote excellence in nursing and healthcare globally through credentialing programs and related services, among which is the ANCC Magnet Recognition Program® (MRP), the "Nobel Prize" of nursing excellence in professional practice environments.

The relationship between shared governance and the MRP program is a synergistic one. Shared governance is a process form of structure for autonomous direct-care nurses to come to the table and share their experiences and secure decision-making power in an organization. Shared governance asks, "What decision have you made lately?" Achieving MRP is a cultural, transformational journey. MRP and shared governance must be a part of the strategic plan for the organization when nursing excellence is the standard of professional practice (Haag-Heitman & George, 2010).

ANCC Magnet Recognition Program® goals

The MRP program has three primary goals:

1. Promote quality of healthcare services in an environment that supports professional nursing practice

2. Identify excellence in the delivery of nursing services to patients/residents

3. Provide a mechanism for the dissemination of "best practices" in nursing services

The journey to MRP shares two central elements with the shared governance process model: cultural enhancements and structural enhancements, as follows.

1. **Cultural enhancements.** The work environment is changed during this process, enabling and empowering nurses at point of care to improve and enhance patient outcomes. The MRP journey will not be successful without a culture of shared decision-making and shared leadership among professional nurses, interprofessional partnerships, and an interdisciplinary team (clinical and administrative) first being in place.

2. **Structural enhancements.** A strategic plan is built around the autonomy of nurses sharing in decision-making and functioning in four primary professional roles: clinical practice, education, research, and administration. Shared governance provides a professional practice environment in which nurses can develop and mature in these roles to effectively enhance the organizational culture.

Benefits of the ANCC Magnet Recognition Program® and shared governance

There are three groups of people already reflecting and building the five Components and 14 Forces of Magnetism into their culture:

1. Those who have implemented shared decision-making, professional nurse autonomy, and the essentials of the 14 Forces of Magnetism and are ready to articulate them

2. Those who are putting the essentials in place and beginning to change the culture before demonstrating it through the application for MRP recognition

3. Those who have chosen to implement the essentials of the culture but may not apply for formal consideration or designation by ANCC

The benefits of MRP are reflected in the effective shared governance described by such nurse researchers as Havens and Aiken (1999) in Figure 8.1:

Figure 8.1	BENEFITS OF DESIGNATION REFLECTED IN SHARED GOVERNANCE

For the patient/client

- Reduced patient mortality
- Reduced patient morbidity
- Increased patient satisfaction
- Increased patient safety
- Decreased "failure to rescue"

For organizations

- Decreased length of stay
- Decreased cost of nursing staff replacement
- Increased opportunity to market institution
- Variable costs of implementation

For nurses

- Lower nurse turnover
- Lower nurse vacancy rates
- Lower nurse "burnout" rates
- Lower nurse emotional exhaustion
- Decreased needlestick injuries
- Better nurse-physician relationships
- Higher nurse satisfaction
- Decreased work-related injuries
- Higher nurse-to-patient ratio
- Decreased medical errors

Shared governance helps those in leadership positions provide a professional practice environment that supports and facilitates direct-care nurse autonomy in:

- Determining education credentials
- Evaluating and writing research
- Writing and/or updating policies and procedures

- Participating in scheduling

- Managing their own competencies

- Providing in-services and continuing education

- Precepting students/new graduates/new employees

- Any other duties they are interested in learning and participating in with their nurse management/ leadership, interdisciplinary team members, and administration

Essentials of nursing excellence

"Eight essentials of magnetism" are evident in every culture of shared governance. They indicate what keeps nurses working in professional practice environments (McClure & Hinshaw, 2002):

1. **Working with clinically competent nurses:** Direct-care nurses participate in identifying their own competencies each year based on what's new, changed, problematic, and high-risk/time-sensitive in the practice environment and verifying how they meet those competencies and collaborating with nurse leaders to identify and verify what organizational competencies also need to be addressed

2. **Good nurse-physician relationships:** Collaborative interprofessional partnerships

3. **Support for education:** Advanced credentialing through facilitation and flexibility of work schedules and resources provided; for example, bringing academic education onto the facility campus out of respect for the nurses' work-life balance needs

4. **Adequate nursing staffing:** Participation in staffing schedules: engagement, involvement, and shared decision-making by staff who are thinking beyond the unit level to the organization as a whole

5. **Concern for the patient is paramount:** Doing what is needed for the staff first (e.g., providing resources and ongoing training to maintain and/or enhance competency) so they can focus all their energy, expertise, and experience on meeting the needs of the patients, the essence of staff-centered, patient-focused, relationship-based care

6. **Nurse autonomy and accountability:** Improving communication and delegation by bringing together partnership, equity, responsibility, authority, ownership, and accountability in shared decision-making and shared leadership in professional practice environments

7. **Supportive nurse manager/supervisor:** The nurse manager or supervisor is the key retention person at the point of care; this role is critical to effective outcomes related to shared decision-making and implementation of the shared governance process model at unit and organizational levels

8. **Control over nursing practice and environment:** In which shared decision-making leads to better patient outcomes and partnerships between patients and healthcare providers

Shared governance pulls everything together and reshapes nursing practice to provide an environment of professional excellence that flows well through the Components and Forces of Magnetism. Through ongoing nursing research and evidences of best practices, nurses excel in shared decision-making at the point of service. They enjoy collegial management and staff partnerships, collaborative practice among all members of the interprofessional and interdisciplinary teams, and accountability-based ownership in issues related to practice, quality, and competence.

Five Components

If the MRP is the Nobel Prize of nursing, the 5 Components and 14 Forces of Magnetism comprise its core and shared governance constitutes their expression in healthcare. The Components and Forces are categories of attributes or outcomes that exemplify nursing excellence evidenced by shared decision-making, partnership, equity, responsibility, accountability, authority, and ownership in professional practice.

The 14 Forces of Magnetism are folded into the 5 Components and are fundamental to determining excellence in the professional nursing practice environment. In 2008, eight domains were also added to describe the model components of magnetism: leadership, resource utilization and development, models that guide practice, safe and ethical practice, autonomous practice, quality processes, research, and outcomes.

MRP is about the journey. The Forces are based on compelling original research (McClure & Hinshaw, 2002) and make it easier to engage nursing leaders and direct-care nurses in the process of shared governance and the MRP journey to nursing excellence—even if they are not going for MRP designation or redesignation.

Components relative to shared governance

TRANSFORMATIONAL LEADERSHIP (Domain: Leadership)

Force 1. Quality of nursing leadership: The chief nursing officer (CNO) is a knowledgeable and strong risk-taker who provides a professional practice environment and philosophy for mutual advocacy and shared decision-making within nursing service among all direct-care nurses and nurse leaders. The CNO sits at the highest decision-making place in the organization—at the senior leadership table—so that all nurses' voices can be heard throughout the organization and their interests represented. The CNO, the ambassador for nursing service, protects nursing leaders and direct-care nurses from political and economic influences that could negatively impact patient care outcomes and/or the professional practice environments.

Force 3. Management style: The CNO and nurse leaders (i.e., managers, directors, supervisors, charge nurses) help direct-care nurses create vision, philosophy, and shared purpose through supportive discussion and reflective practice. Feedback is valued and communicated at all levels of the organization as appropriate. Direct-care nurse leaders are visible, accessible, and committed to working closely with the interdisciplinary team and other direct-care providers. Nurse leaders provide support, encouragement, resources, boundaries, and protection through the shared governance organizational management process model in matters of professional nursing practice, quality, and competence. The management style is grounded in transformational, servant leadership and shared decisional processes with an outcome of shared leadership the goal for all direct-care nurses.

STRUCTURAL EMPOWERMENT (Domains: Resource utilization and development)

Force 2. Organizational structure: The macrosystem has decentralized, flat organizational structures, creating a sense of partnership, equity, accountability, and ownership within professional practice environments. Typically, the CNO reports directly to the CEO and serves at the executive level of the organization. MRP has no criteria for how the organizational structure should or should not look. However, there must be a structure and process of some kind in place that is dynamic and responsive to change. A formal structure is critical to manage nurses' involvement through a representative model. Every organization develops its models and cultures differently but includes strategic planning, shared decision-making, and staff responsiveness. The organization demonstrates strong nursing representation in council and committee structures and through a functioning and productive system of shared decisional processes.

Force 4. Personnel policies and programs: Direct-care nurses are involved in decision-making about budgets, schedules, salaries, competencies, resources, and practice. For example, they should be familiar with budgets and their roles and responsibilities related to organizational and unit stewardship. Salaries and benefits are competitive with community standards with opportunities for advancement and promotions, awards, and/or bonuses for exceptional services. Job descriptions, written in partnership by nurses and representatives from human resources, reflect the characteristics of the essentials of nursing excellence grounded in the tenets and scopes of professional nursing practice (e.g., direct-care nurses, clinical nurse leaders, clinical nurse educators, nurse managers, and advanced practice nurses).

A best practice in participative scheduling

Creative and flexible staffing models and schedules accommodate the many demands direct-care nurses experience on their time and attention at work and at home. Increased patient acuities and workloads require negotiation and shared decision-making at the point of service to maximize staff satisfaction. For example, one innovative group of direct-care nurses worked with their nurse manager to restructure their shift hours. The unit council studied the possibilities, conferred with other staff and direct-care nurses regarding the proposed changes in shift rotations, and successfully demonstrated how improved patient care outcomes could positively support their proposal. After further negotiation with leadership and human resources, the unit council informed staff they could pilot a change in their 12-hour shift rotations to 3 a.m. to 3 p.m. and 3 p.m. to 3 a.m. for six months. The new schedule resulted in a more enthusiastic and committed staff, fewer call-ins, the expected improvements in patient satisfaction and care outcomes, and a deeper respect for nursing leadership and the process of shared decision-making.

Force 10. Community and the healthcare organization: Healthcare providers build relationships within and among all types of healthcare and community organizations. They develop strong partnerships supportive of positive patient outcomes and the health of the local communities they serve. Nurses in shared governance recognize and embrace their responsibilities to support community outreach activities that result in nursing service and the organization being seen as strong, positive, and productive community citizens. This is accomplished through community collaboration, positive outcomes from collaborations, and allocating and using appropriate resources as needed.

A best practice in community outreach

Paul F. Sink, Jr., nursing education coordinator for the Community Living Center at James A. Haley VA Healthcare System in Florida, coordinates the continuing nursing education provided for a workshop on hurricane awareness for Tampa and surrounding communities each year. He is part of a multidisciplinary team of healthcare providers, safety specialists, and subject matter experts working to help the citizens remain safe, calm, and ready during the many hurricanes and tropical storms they struggle to endure each hurricane season, whether storms come or only threaten.

Force 12. Image of nursing: Ask direct-care nurses to describe what MRP and shared governance mean to them. Build and expand the image of nursing within the organization and community. Nursing service's contributions are recognized and rewarded. Other members of the healthcare team characterize nursing services as essential to the organization and integral to the overall well-being of patients. The direct-care nurses' voice is heard and respected in the governing councils, in other departments and divisions, and in their nurse-physician and interdisciplinary team member relationships, effectively influencing system-wide processes.

A best practice in building influence and the image of nurses

Sandra F. Law, clinical nurse educator at the Bay Pines VA Healthcare System in Florida, facilitated the development of professional nurse portfolios with template dividers for distribution to every certified nurse in the organization during Nurses' Week 2010. Prior to the celebration, photographs of each certified nurse were taken and put on a colorful PowerPoint® slide, complete with credentials, title, and the specialty or specialties of certification. All of the pictures were printed and became the cover for each nurse's portfolio. These pictures were also folded into a looped program shown during a formal recognition ceremony held during Nurses' Week. Invitations and announcements went out organizationwide. The CEO, the chief of staff, the CNO, nurse leaders, and other service leaders, as well as many of the nursing staff and their friends and colleagues, attended. Each certified nurse was presented his or her portfolio by the CNO and had his/her picture taken with the CNO and executive leaders. Throughout this incredible program honoring the significant accomplishments of these exceptional nurses, the program with each and every one of their pictures and accomplishments played in the background. After, one direct-care nurse brought his portfolio to the registration table and, with tears in his eyes, thanked those present for the "best Nurses' Week gift I have ever gotten!"

Best practices in nursing professional development

Contributing author: Yvonne Brookes, RN, corporate director of the Department of Clinical Learning at Baptist Health South Florida, Miami.

Shared governance is a new concept for many direct-care nurses. We are just beginning to change our culture. The Department of Clinical Learning leaders and clinical educators at Baptist Health South Florida work with direct-care nurses to help them go as far as they choose to in their professional development through transformational leadership and specialized practice in nursing professional development. Ms. Brooks identified some of the many ways this is accomplished, assuring patients and colleagues of the best possible care outcomes.

The Department of Clinical Learning provides evidence-based nursing education to foster clinical and service excellence, quality outcomes, patient safety, and research. Clinical educators have created a learning environment at point of care for direct-care nurses to develop and enhance their professional competencies, critical thinking and clinical judgment skills, and interprofessional collaborative relationships through such activities as:

- Employee engagement

- Clinical partnerships

- Team-based nurse competency validations

- Expanded simulation learning methods

- An RN residency program

- Specialty certifications and awards

- Accreditation of continuing nursing education through the ANCC's Accreditation Program

- Investigational Review Board–approved research studies (i.e., outcome measures to monitor program effectiveness: self-efficacy, knowledge attainment, and influence on practice pre- and postprogressive care academy; principal investigators Donna Lee Wilson, RN, MSN, CCRN, and Denise Haughton, RN, MSN)

- Orientation of staff to organization and unit

- Continuing and mandatory education at unit levels

- In-service planning and education

- The Critical Care Academy

- The Progressive Care Academy

- Multiple preceptor and mentoring programs

Between October 2009 and September 2010, more than 19,800 participants attended over 259,100 learner hours of in-person educational offerings facilitated and/or provided by the Department of Clinical Learning staff. These hours do not reflect the countless additional hours of education and in-services that occurred at the point of care by the unit-level council members, individual nurses, clinical educators, preceptors, and other clinicians in this extraordinary evidence of best practice related to a commitment to excellence in nursing professional development.

EXEMPLARY PROFESSIONAL PRACTICE (Domains: Models that guide practice, safe and ethical practice, autonomous practice, and quality processes)

Force 5. Professional models of care: Although this can be a confusing Force for some, it is important for nurses to know the differences between professional practice models of care and care delivery systems. Professional models of care look at which nursing theorists are used in the organization (i.e., Benner, Neuman, King, or Orem). Can nurses talk about them in the following ways? (1) Who are they? (2) What are theorists needed for—what is their purpose? Professional care models provide a theoretical foundation on which to build research and contrasts and comparisons. They are the basis of the discipline of nursing. Because there is no one theory that covers all patient populations with their unique needs, organizations usually have several theorists that blend into the conceptual framework and reflect values and philosophies of each nursing service.

MRP defines a *professional practice model* as "the driving force of nursing care" (*The Magnet Model Components and Sources of Evidence: Magnet Recognition Program®*, 2008, p. 44). Shared governance practice councils delineate the models of care and make sure there is evidence hardwired into the organization and nurses have adequate resources to accomplish desired patient care outcomes.

A *care delivery system* is defined as "a system for the provision of care that delineates the nurses' authority and accountability for clinical decision-making and outcomes" (*The Magnet Model Components and Sources of Evidence: Magnet Recognition Program®*, 2008, p. 38). For example, team nursing is a care delivery system. It is not a conceptual model of care. Rocchiccioli and Tilbury (1998) describe eight care delivery systems: functional nursing, team nursing, primary nursing, primary-team nursing, total patient care, modular nursing, differentiated practice, and case management.

Nurses are accountable for their own professional practice models and the systems of care delivery selected for nursing service. Shared governance provides a process structure for assessments, strategic change, and ongoing evaluation of patient outcomes and care delivery systems that promote professionalism, accountability, evidence-based practice, adaptation to regulatory needs, and a staffing system reflective of patient needs. Models of nursing care (i.e., the relationship-based care model) give direct-care nurses the responsibility, authority, and accountability needed to provide and coordinate patient care at the point of service (Wright, 2002). Nurses need to know they are all practicing under the same standards.

Force 8. Consultation and resources: This Force is about cataloging local and/or national speakers brought in for training, nursing grand rounds, clinical nurse specialists (in consultative roles), experts and expertise available within the organization or made available by bringing in consultants, and taking field trips to other facilities to review and/or learn about best practices in nursing. The organization and nursing service provide adequate resources, support, and opportunities for these activities.

Force 9. Autonomy is one of the fundamental principles of shared governance: Direct-care nurses within the organization govern their own practice and share in making decisions affecting practice, quality, and competence. They partner with other healthcare providers and patients to deliver care at point of service. Nurse leaders facilitate nurses' success by providing the resources, support, encouragement, and boundaries they need to dispense patient-focused care.

Force 11. Nurses as teachers: Nurses educate, precept, coach, orient, and mentor other nurses, students, and patients within the organization. They get involved in the lifelong learning of others, both inside and outside their communities. Students from a variety of clinical and academic programs are welcomed, supported, and engaged in the organization. Affiliation agreements and contractual arrangements are mutually beneficial. In a shared governance practice setting, direct-care nurses are supported by leadership

---

Best practices in autonomous practice through unit councils

Contributing author: Solimar Figueroa, MSN, MHA, BSN, RN, CNOR, clinical educator, Department of Clinical Learning, Baptist Health South Florida, Miami

Baptist Health South Florida piloted implementation of autonomous direct-care nurse unit-level competency assessments on a medical surgical unit utilizing their unit councils (i.e., unit practice councils [UPC]). They chose to adapt the Wright model (2005) and Swihart's Competency Decision Worksheet (see Appendix 28) for the pilot. Previously, competency validations had been done through biannual skills fairs. Attendance in these skills fairs has been mandated for compliance.

The Wright model was presented to unit staff at the UPC monthly meeting. They were provided definitions and descriptions of the following:

- Competency assessment, purpose, and benefits

- Roles and delineation of internal and external stakeholders

- Processes involved in the transition to this approach for competency validation

---

Best practices in autonomous practice through unit councils (cont.)

- Selecting unit-level competencies based on what is new, changed, problematic, and/or high-risk/time-sensitive

- Training staff in peer verification, monitoring processes and activities, and reporting structures for outcomes

The proposal for implementation of unit-level competency validations reflected an organizational culture shift. The newly delineated roles of the stakeholders for the pilot involving the manager, nurse clinicians, and point-of-care staff were clearly and distinctly articulated to facilitate more successful outcomes. The unit-level competency model promoted accountability and best practices through the active engagement of the UPC members and direct-care nurses.

The UPC members disseminated the information presented to the council to the rest of the staff by following "trees" of communication. Each UPC member has a corresponding tree with between five and 10 assigned staff members. The staff received information from the UPC and then communicated back through their UPC representatives which competencies they identified as important for them. The unit council collected the information, and UPC members selected the competencies for the unit and determined the duration of each competency cycle (e.g., once, ongoing/annual, quarterly).

The collaboration among the manager, staff, and nurse clinicians in establishing the unit-level competencies was a phenomenal success based on the reported unit outcomes from the pilot. For example, the peer verification process embedded in the Wright model empowered the nurses to take charge of their professional practice. Nurses were trained how to give reflective feedback to their colleagues as they selected and validated identified competencies at the unit level. This collegial, peer-to-peer approach promoted better communication among staff, encouraging them to help one another during the selection of competencies and validation processes. This gives the staff more autonomy in their own professional practice, competence, and quality, which contributes to improved patient care outcomes, satisfaction, safety, and compliance. It is one of the many best practices found at Baptist Health South Florida.

and expected to serve as educators and/or teachers to ensure the foundation for quality of care, a direct-care nurse domain, and ongoing competencies. Nurse development and mentoring programs prepare staff preceptors to work with all levels of students.

Nurses in all positions serve as faculty and preceptors for students and new employees. Direct-care nurses provide patient and family education, clinical and leadership development, in-services, and scholarly initiatives.

Best practice of nurses as unit educators (UE) in shared governance

The UE is generally a direct-care nurse who is responsible for assessing, planning, coordinating, and evaluating the educational needs of the nursing staff at the unit level. The UE works closely with the unit council members, nursing staff, and the nurse manager to identify educational programs and activities that develop and maintain staff competencies. The UE helps direct-care nurses provide quality care for the unique patient population on his or her assigned units by facilitating a continuous learning environment. Other activities may include the following:

- Identify in-service education needs of staff with the assistance and support of other nurse clinicians

- Coordinate in-service programs with direct-care nurses and others

- Schedule speakers for varied in-services based on assessed needs

- Network with other UEs to share information and provide cross-training when appropriate

- Publicize centralized nursing education learning activities

- Maintain accurate records of individual staff members' attendance at in-service programs, mandatory reviews, and external learning events

- Enter training data into the hospital education tracking system

- Help the nursing staff retrieve the data whenever needed

Each month, UEs may attend meetings to discuss their roles and responsibilities and how their work fits into the overarching strategic plan for continuing nursing education and staff development within the whole organization. They hold a great deal of respect, autonomy, and mutual accountability with the nursing staff because they are helping nurses ensure excellence in nursing care at point of service.

Force 13. Interdisciplinary relationships: Shared governance creates a forum for direct-care nurses, interprofessional partners (nurses, physicians, and pharmacists), and interdisciplinary team members to develop and enhance mutual respect, knowledge, competence, and a platform for essential and meaningful contributions toward quality clinical outcomes. Collaborative working relationships within and among the disciplines are actively cultivated and valued.

NEW KNOWLEDGE, INNOVATIONS, AND IMPROVEMENTS (Domain: Research)

Force 7. Quality improvement (QI): QI is the process that advances the quality of care and services within the organization. QI focuses on operational effectiveness and clinical processes and outcomes.

Best practices of QI through nursing case study investigations (CSI) in shared governance

Contributing author: Michelle Jans, MSN, RN-BC, nurse manager, Bay Pines VA Healthcare System, Bay Pines, FL

The nursing CSI is a process for analyzing the events around patient outcomes that resulted in either near misses and/or medical errors of varying degrees in practice settings. Each month, quarterly, or as needed, case studies are developed by direct-care nurses around real incidents identified through root cause analyses, incident reports, or tagged by nursing leadership and/or direct-care nurses as potential learning opportunities to improve patient outcomes. Direct-care nurses from all shifts and inpatient units identify "clues" to the underlying problem(s) that may have changed the patient's outcome if they had been recognized earlier. Using a detectivelike method of inquiry, nurses are able to uncover critical and often-missed clues to help them see the bigger picture and solve the case to complete the following:

- Diagnose learning needs

- Implement advanced assessment skills, critical thinking, and evidence-based practice

- Discover limited and/or incomplete data within policies that would help provide a more appropriate clinical pathway to the presenting clinical picture

- Increase communication and collaboration among interdisciplinary team members

- Improve documentation in content and context

- Enhance professional practice skills (organization, prioritization, delegation, problem solving)

- Engage in open and honest peer review

Through shared exploration and problem solving, the nursing CSI has become an integral forum for nurses to achieve a greater level of excellence by way of careful consideration of the evidences in practice, evaluation of the clues along the way, and successful solutions to the case at hand.

EMPIRICAL QUALITY OUTCOMES (Domain: Outcomes)

Force 6. Quality of care and quality improvement (Force 7) are about structure and outcomes: Quality of care is about the effectiveness of the system to support nursing and patient care. Direct-care nurses engaged in shared governance make meaningful decisions about quality practice at the point of service. They are responsible for providing evidence-based care grounded in research that facilitates improved patient care outcomes in quality of care and QI in decisions related to practice, quality, and competence.

Empirical quality outcomes related to quality of care and QI are best realized in environments of care with shared governance. Quality assurance and performance improvement are process-driven approaches, usually with specific steps for design, development, production or service, and evaluation or verification (i.e., performance measures), that guide definitions and achieve or exceed identified goals. Direct-care nurses participate in quality practice at the point of service through shared governance at unit and organizational levels.

The Relationship Between Shared Governance and the ISO 9001:2008 Quality Management System

Contributing author: Dawn Barrowman, ARNP, regional nurse with the VHA Office of Clinical Consultation and Compliance; and Colonel, U. S. Army Reserves

A corporation is a living organism; it has to continue to shed its skin. Methods have to change. Focus has to change. Values have to change. The sum total of those changes is transformation.

– Andrew Grove

Over the past two decades, the military and U.S. Department of Veterans Affairs (VA) have expanded and reconceptualized nurse roles as part of restructuring services and resdesign of systems to meet the growing needs of veterans. Seeking better ways to operate more efficiently and effectively, they recognized how critical nurses are in reducing and preventing medication errors and infections, in establishing and maintaining quality of services and care, as well as transitioning patients from hospital to home, especially when nurses lead these efforts in collaboration with interprofessional partners and interdisciplinary team members (Institutes of Medicine, 2011; *www1.va.gov/health*)

Additionally, with so many agencies surveying and auditing performance and processes in healthcare organizations today, there is a growing need for nurses in all environments of care to gain a broader knowledge of national and international standards with application to practice (i.e., The Joint Commission [TJC], the National Database for Nursing Quality Indicators, ANCC [i.e., MRP, accreditation, certifications], and the ISO). Within the context of excellence in healthcare through long-term growth and change, the goal is to exceed customer and organizational expectations through measurable and accountable processes. To do this, it is important for nurses to understand and use models of process-based quality management systems (QMS) within their organizations to effect change and continual quality improvements.

The ISO

The standards from the ISO are not prescriptive, determining that all things should be uniform or the same. They do encourage equality in quality, purpose, expectations, approach, and achievement. Organizations conforming to the requirements of an ISO standard could be considered equals in quality management even though they will not operationalize those standards or principles in exactly the same way. Much like organizations that conform to TJC standards, the ANCC MRP and accreditation criteria, and/or the Baldrige National Quality Program criteria, the similarities between and among ISO organizations are evident in:

+ Consistent service

+ Customer satisfaction

+ Continuous improvement

Since 1947, ISO has published more than 18,500 international standards with roots in engineering, construction, agriculture, medical devices, and now, information technology developments. ISO does not include requirements specific to other management systems (i.e., those particular to occupational health and safety management, environmental management, or risk management) but does enable an organization to align and integrate its own QMS with related management system requirements.

ISO is a nongovernmental organization headquartered in Geneva, Switzerland, that bridges public and private sectors. It has a global community of member bodies. ISO uses technical committees representing their sectors of expertise to prepare standards with international application and use. Each member body votes to accept standards that apply to the organizations, people, products, and services of that nation.

What's in a name? Much. This global organization required an equally global name. A translation of the words *International Organization for Standardization* yields different acronyms and initialisms in different languages ("IOS" in English, "OIN" in French for *Organisation Internationale de Normalization*, or "OIE" in Spanish for *Organización Internacional para la Estandarización*). Therefore, its founders chose to add a short, all-purpose name for branding their work: ISO, derived from the Greek *isos*, meaning equal. Whatever the country or language, the short form of the organization's name is always ISO (*www.iso.org/iso/about/discover-iso_isos-name.htm*).

Presently, the use of ISO standards, clauses, and principles inside the healthcare delivery arena, system, facilities, and support systems proffers an open market. The QMS within ISO is designed to incorporate standardization of process and procedures, products, organizational structure, and execution of services. The intent is standardization with site-specific customization to the facility, area, service, or location to streamline the workload, to improve the effectiveness of the organization, then to enhance the efficiency of it (American National Standards Institute, ISO, & ASQ-E, 2008).

How does ISO compare to TJC?

The TJC, established in 1975, has long been known as the "gold standard" for quality among healthcare providers. The voluntary accreditation process through TJC provides tools and consultative advice to improve business operations. Accreditation and/or certification is a process separate from the healthcare organization, usually nongovernmental, in which TJC assesses the organization to determine if it meets a set of standard requirements to improve quality of care, as well as offering brand recognition.

The Joint Commission International Accreditation operates in conjunction with international healthcare organizations, public health agencies, health ministries, and other entities to improve the quality of patient care in their nations while voluntarily obliging to specific legal, religious, and cultural factors within a country.

If ISO standards are not Joint Commission, what are they?

ISO 9000, a family of standards relating to the QMS within an organization, provides general information about the QMS requirements for improving processes. The ISO 9001, a later version of ISO 9000, is also a business management system in that it speaks to how an organization does business as well.

The use of ISO standards within a healthcare facility, setting, or scope of practice stands to realize cost savings while empowering employee satisfaction. An example for use in military medicine speaks to the professional credentialing process of providers within all military treatment facilities and outside U.S. Department of Defense (DoD) entities to standardize the process. The system currently in place may be similar; however, duplication and redundancies are present in every military facility and branch of military service, as well as civilian-supported military entities. Military installations have become joint bases and operate in every realm of the DoD to include the VA system with some interoperability. ISO, coupled with shared governance, offers nurses an opportunity to streamline processes, reduce variances, and eliminate redundancies through shared leadership around professional practice and credentialing.

How does ISO work? ISO promotes adoption of a process approach to develop, implement, and improve the effectiveness of a QMS for enhancing satisfaction by meeting customer requirements. Shared governance provides a structure in which nurses implement and/or maintain a process approach for managing quality to drive innovation and continual improvements in services and organizational stewardship (i.e., business practices and fiscal responsibilities) at point of service.

The Shewhart Cycle (plan, do, check, act [PDCA]) is an effective process-based method for establishing, tracking, and monitoring quality and improvements at the unit level. It is a straightforward approach that can be applied to all processes. Direct-care nurses use PDCA to analyze existing conditions and methods for providing safe, effective, efficient patient care in all practice settings. The Shewhart Cycle was developed by Dr. W. Edwards Deming and named for Walter Shewhart, who discussed the concept in his book *Statistical Method from the Viewpoint of Quality Control* (1939). One of the more common QI tools in healthcare, PDCA consists of four steps easily implemented through unit councils at points of service:

- **Plan:** Identify and establish goals/objectives and processes needed to deliver the desired outcomes

- **Do:** Implement the process(es) developed

- **Check:** Monitor, measure, and evaluate the implemented process by testing the results against the predetermined goals or objectives

- **Act:** Take actions necessary to continually improve process performance and patient care outcomes

Principles of ISO 9001 and the shared governance process

The QMS, process resdesign, and eight principles for ISO 9001 and how they compare to the shared governance process model are important concepts for establishing and advancing quality improvement monitors, measures, and outcomes. ISO is a QMS of processes, not one of blame. ISO process-based systems:

- Provide benchmarks for continual improvement, complementing other management systems, products, and services

- Provide effective and efficient control of processes by management, which is:

    – Leading, directing, and controlling to achieve a specified outcome

    – Planning groups of activities to be carried out

    – Coordinating activities and use of resources within the organization to meet specified goals

- Provide for self-evaluation by the organization:

    – Cost reduction (profit enhancer)

    – Continual improvement

    – Effective management control

- Reduce cost of poor performance and systems redundancies

- Identify weaker areas of the system for improvement and/or resdesign

- Provide an environment for consistency and predictability of output to meet customer, applicable regulatory, and stakeholder requirements

- Clearly define roles, responsibilities, and information flow by process

- Support nurse involvement and ownership of processes

- Validate nurses' competencies in their tasks

- Increase stakeholder (leaders, nurses, patients, and others) confidence

ISO-based standards, then, provide a foundation for the development of a management structure in which shared governance facilitates movement from micromanagement to leadership through shared decision-making and continuous quality improvement. Engagement with nurses helps define the right amount of management control to ensure an effective and efficient quality system of shared leadership at the point of service. The most successfully designed and implemented management structures involve top management (i.e., within the management system scope) and the people performing the tasks and activities, especially at points of service.

As people (e.g., direct-care nurses, advanced practice nurses, nurse generalists), technologies, environments of care, and customers (i.e., patient populations) change, so too must quality management control systems change. Measurement and review systems are needed to stay abreast of the changes and maintain the right amount of management control.

ISO 9001 is a quality and business management system that can provide organizations a process-based approach to managing daily operations and supporting relationships with stakeholders (i.e., patients, healthcare providers, and suppliers). It helps nurses define and guide the right amount of management control within the context of eight quality management principles for sustained performance improvements. These eight principles (with adaptations to healthcare added in brackets) include:

1. **Customer focus [the patient]:** Organizations depend on their customers and so need to understand current and future needs, striving to meet and exceed customer requirements and expectations (e.g., primary care, patient-centered care, medical home models, clinical nurse leaders)

2. **Leadership:** Establish unit of purpose and direction of organization [service and unit]; create and maintain internal environments in which nurses can become fully involved in achieving the goals and objectives of the organization and the nursing service:

   – Leadership begins with the mission (how organizations define the reasons for their existence) and identifying who the customer is (customer focus and leadership)

   – Top management communicates the mission and where they want to direct the organization (vision) to the nurses (employees) to engage them in the process (leadership and involvement of people)

3. **Involvement of people:** People at all levels—nurses at all levels—are the essence of the organization and their full involvement enables their abilities to be used to benefit the organization (i.e., shared governance and engagement)

4. **Process approach:** A desired result or outcome is achieved more efficiently when activities and related resources are managed as a process:

   – The organization can involve its people to define the processes in support of the mission and vision (process approach, involvement of people, and leadership)

- Processes, when connected, form the management system defined to meet the organization's mission and vision (system approach to management, leadership, and customer focus)

5. **System approach to management:** Identifying, understanding, and managing interrelated processes as a system contributes to the organization's effectiveness and efficiency in achieving its objectives

6. **Continual improvement** of the organization's overall performance should be a permanent objective or goal of the organization:

   - Once the management system is defined, the organization can identify the measurements needed to continually improve in satisfying patients, nurses, and other customers (system approach to management, factual approach to decision-making, continual improvement, and customer focus)

   - These measurements can have significant impact on quality when direct-care nurses participate at the unit level through shared governance activities at point of service

7. **Factual approach to decision-making:** Effective decisions are based on the analysis of data and information [and evidenced in changes in practice to improve patient safety and care outcomes]

8. **Mutually beneficial supplier relationships:** An organization and its suppliers are interdependent and have a mutually beneficial relationship that enhances the ability of both to create value (e.g., surgical suppliers, administrative and clinical supplies, products, and services related to healthcare):

   - It is mutually beneficial to involve suppliers to help with the organization's customer focus (mutually beneficial supplier relationship and customer focus)

   - Examples of such relationships (mutually beneficial supplier relationship and customer focus) include the following:

     ◦ When an equipment supplier provides training to nurses and staff members on how to safely and effectively use the equipment

     ◦ When suppliers and customers share information and data to improve products and services

Healthcare organizations generally define their customers as their patients, implementing patient-centered policies and standards to guide care and services. The purpose of quality management is to ensure products and services achieve customer (patient) satisfaction through customer (patient)-oriented processes. This is best achieved at the points of service through engaged nurses and effective team members. Unit-level councils provide a structure for identifying, monitoring, measuring, and evaluating quality of services and care to facilitate continual performance and process improvement in all practice settings.

Leadership and nurse managers create an environment that fully engages nurses, one in which a QMS can operate effectively and in which transformative leadership is demonstrated in the following ways:

+ Through actions and follow-through (communication and task completion)

+ Direction/guidance provided

+ Tools and resources to be successful provided

+ Flexibility—able to adopt, adapt, or abandon; ability to adapt and adjust plans wherever needed (ISO Consultants for Healthcare, 2010)

The ANCC established their Accreditation Program in 1974 to recognize organizations (or components of organizations) that provide high-quality continuing education for nurses at all levels. In 2007, ANCC received ISO 9001:2008 certification in all of their credentialing programs, including professional services rendered in the administration of the MRP for excellence in nursing in healthcare organizations, the Accreditation Program for excellence in continuing nursing education, Pathway to Excellence® Program for excellence in healthcare organizations, and the Certification Program.

ANCC noted how organizations implementing an ISO 9001:2008 QMS usually achieved important benefits (i.e., a more organized operating environment, effective and efficient operations, improved employee morale, increased staff engagement, and improved customer satisfaction). Implementation of an ISO 9001 QMS helps to build a strong quality culture of ownership, accountability, and overall improved performance. Roles and responsibilities are clearly articulated, processes are defined and documented, and an overall culture of standardization, consistency, and quality results are realized through shared governance and professional autonomy. In achieving ISO certification, ANCC effectively demonstrated that all of their programs, products, and services are based on uniform principles, policies, and standards (adapted from ANCC, 2011).

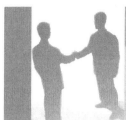

TIPS FOR SUCCESS

LEARNING OBJECTIVES

After reading this chapter, the participant should be able to:

- Describe 10 tips for success when implementing shared governance

"Come to the edge," he said.
They said, "We are afraid."
"Come to the edge," he said.
They came. He pushed them ... and they flew.

– *Guillaume Appollinaire*

Best Practices Shared by Direct-Care Nurses, Team Leaders, and Other Organizations

This book was written to take some of the guesswork out of the various structures and processes behind shared governance, to provide some basic tools for establishing and developing shared governance at the unit and governance council levels. Throughout these chapters and sections, a number of strategies, case examples, and best practices have been provided to make the daily operations of shared governance meaningful and successful. This chapter is a brief listing of additional tips and ideas to further entice you to enjoy the shared governance process and your journey in reshaping to transform professional nursing practice for today and tomorrow. The future of nursing depends on where you go from here.

1. Schedule a daylong retreat away from the organization to prepare organizational and nursing leaders to implement shared governance. Discuss the role shared governance plays in the American Nurses Credentialing Center Magnet Recognition Program® (MRP) journey. Have subject matter experts present topic discussions on specific points: leadership, shared governance partners, steering committee formation, design team for the shared governance model, a business case for MRP and shared governance, and roles of direct-care nurses and the multidisciplinary team members.

2. Create expectations for staff contributions, beginning in the new employee orientation and continuing throughout their careers.

3. Communicate, communicate, communicate! Have a nursing town hall meeting at least once per quarter to facilitate open communication among nursing staff and leaders.

4. Administer the Index of Professional Nursing Governance surveys and see how your organization "measures up"—help build the repository of information on the efficacy and value of shared governance in healthcare settings.

5. Visit the *Online Journal of Issues in Nursing* to view articles like "Shared governance: Is it a model for nurses to gain control over their practice?" at *www.nursingworld.org/MainMenuCategories/ANAMarketplace/ANAPeriodicals/OJIN/wJournalTopics/SharedGovernance.aspx*.

6. Use journal clubs, for example, to bring nursing research to the bedside and engage direct-care nurses in evidence-based practice for developing and implementing advanced decision-making and critical thinking (see Appendix 17, a guide for enhancing practice through journal clubs).

7. Let direct-care nurses meet each year to review organizational competencies and unit/area needs and determine which competencies they will focus on for that year (high-risk/time-sensitive, changed, problematic, and/or new).

8. Train every registered nurse on each unit/area to be charge or lead nurse. Rotate the role and responsibilities to encourage leadership skills development and shared decision-making among all team members.

9 Involve all staff members in preparing and adapting their schedules to accommodate the needs of their work area. Open staffing to flexible schedules and peer-negotiated days off. Nurse leaders should only step in if there are irreconcilable differences, stalemates, or to help nurses with the process. Responsibility here, as in other areas of shared governance, must be coupled with appropriate levels of authority and accountability to be successful.

10 Communicate the process, expectations, roles, and responsibilities for nurses engaged in shared decision-making throughout the organization, not just on the units/areas.

11 Address management and leadership styles in the shared governance process model selected.

12 Make sure all nurse executives, directors, supervisors, and managers are trained and engaged in the shared governance process model development before bringing staff into the mix. Otherwise, the nursing leaders may become confused or uncomfortable and sabotage the work before it even begins.

13 Recognize and celebrate those direct-care nurses who represent their peers and patients on the shared governance councils and in the community. Support them through creative staffing, "surprise" celebrations, quiet encouragements, and provision of whatever resources they need to be successful.

14 Prepare, support, and encourage nurse change champions to help lead strategic change and facilitate the implementation of shared governance and the MRP journey.

15 Display unit exhibits, bulletin boards, and other learning events, staff activities, and staff celebrations and/or awards.

16 Create an organizational "who's who" of your best practice nurses, MRP champions, and hospital heroes to share with the organization and community.

17 Celebrate every milestone and moment of excellence completed along the way to organizational change through shared governance.

18 Attend workshops and seminars on shared governance, MRP, and leadership in professional practice.

19 Network with organizations that have implemented shared governance successfully or are just beginning their journey (several have been referenced in this book). Share best practices with them.

20 Once shared governance is fully implemented and the organizational culture is ready, begin the MRP journey.

21 **Share success stories peer to peer, unit to unit, area to area, staff to leaders, leaders to staff. Select one each month to present at town hall meetings, leadership meetings, in-services, cafeterias, and elevators. Shared governance takes on a life of its own when it becomes real and exciting to those participating in it. We generate creative and innovative ideas, encouragement, and enthusiasm from one another's experiences.**

22 Use the unit councils to identify what is needed for direct-care nurses to be successful in their own microsystems (i.e., engaged nurse managers and direct supervisors; knowledge and mentoring in the principles, characteristics, and tools of shared governance for staff and managers; and a commitment from the organization, from all of nursing service, and specifically from all members at the unit levels that shared governance is the organizational management structure for how nurses "do business" every day).

23 **Prepare, educate, and support managers about the implications affecting staff ownership and management support. For many, this is a new way of managing their nurses. Precept and mentor them in their roles, responsibilities, and accountabilities in shared decisional processes.**

24 This is key: Practicing in a shared governance organizational management infrastructure and professional practice model is not optional. Ownership, engagement, and active participation in the professional communities of practice are essential and must not be by invitation. If participation in shared governance is optional, than the option eventually becomes the rule (see Chapter 4 for more on what occurs when optional participation is allowed).

25 **Take the time needed to build an effective, efficient, safe infrastructure that supports sustainable behaviors related to ownership, autonomous practice, and shared decision-making at the unit level and beyond.**

26 Remember to look at the "big picture"—think long-term and avoid short-term fixes, decisions, and actions; pay very close attention to the details in the big picture. Participate in strategic planning at the macrosystem (organization) level to better plan and engage all stakeholders at the meso- (nursing service) and microsystems (unit) levels. Alignment of mission, goals, and work now and over time is critical to the success of all three.

27 "Never forget: Caring for others moves us quickly beyond the practical. When a care provider crosses the threshold of a patient and family's door, he or she crosses a border, moving from the world of practical preparation into that of a personal healing relationship in which everything he or she does is in service to the patient. This border crossing brings care providers into the patient's and family's world—a world about which they know little—and within which they must tread with great humility." – Jayne Felgen

28 Learn how to fail forward and turn mistakes and missteps into building blocks (Maxwell, 2007). Frequently reenergize staff and shared governance champions by looking at what is happening not as a failure but as a point of stepping back to renew and refine some structures and processes, to build a stronger framework for the development of meaningful and sustainable professional practice within a shared governance model which exemplifies it.

29 "Many companies define [human resources] as being solely responsible for attraction, motivation, and retention. Our approach has always been to entrust our great [nurses] with that responsibility." – Elizabeth Barrett

30 Think proactive, not reactive. Stop and take a deep breath before moving forward, speaking, or acting. Ask questions. Step back and look at the situation or event from a new perspective. This is how a transformational leader approaches problems, crises, and other disasters, both potential and real.

31 Create, maintain, and share professional portfolios. Follow one another's professional activities: presentations, academic advancements, certifications, and contributions through professional organizations, affiliations, committees, advisory boards, and other accomplishments. Encourage and support one another through shared possibilities and opportunities.

32 Solicit and apply best practices from other people, units, departments, and organizations.

33 Volunteer with enthusiasm! Take action!

34 Identify a unit council facilitator to coordinate council activities; work closely with the nurse manager and direct-care nurses to determine what activities, projects, and tasks are workable for change, development, or implementation; identify unit issues/concerns to bring before the council; and communicate issues/concerns/outcomes to all direct-care nurses and staff on all shifts.

35 Create a quarterly report of activities, accomplishments, outcomes, and celebrations to record and communicate progress in improving and advancing professional nursing practice, quality, and competency through shared governance and influencing decisions across the organization.

36 Take classes and courses not directly job-related (e.g., crucial conversations, how to do stand-up comedy, writing for everyone, blogging for exercise, and so on) to relax and energize creative thinking—and to provide more interesting icebreakers for unit council meetings.

37 Collect and share professional journals, newsletters, and magazines.

38 "Share knowledge freely and ask others to do the same, ideally in small digestible chunks."
– Scott Adams

39 "Make 'teaching' a part of everyone's job description. Reward those who do a good job of communicating useful information to staff on all shifts, including off-tours." – Adams, 1996, p. 322

40 Listen actively (invest in what is being said) to learn from others and adapt to include their perspectives. Teams need active listening to consider any issue or point of discussion from all sides and make clear and accurate decisions together.

41 Everyone's job is important. Engage each person at the unit level and beyond in the mission, values, and goals of the organization and each practice setting. Celebrate every contribution—large and small—to the safety and care of patients and their families.

42 Learn from students' and new employees' experiences and skills. Bring them into the unit council as soon as possible. Do not lose the opportunities they bring to the table. They usually have a wealth of information, questions, and a perspective that can advance practice in new and interesting ways.

43 Be open and available to one another.

44 When participating in peer review, give feedback all along the way. Identify both positive accomplishments and opportunities to improve and grow as they occur and share them then. There should be no surprises at evaluation time.

SHARED GOVERNANCE, SECOND EDITION

45 Let people make mistakes—as long as they do not jeopardize patient safety. This is an excellent way to impact learning and influence change.

46 Take five to 10 minutes before each unit council meeting to receive information, questions, ideas, requests, and/or cautions from nurse managers. Sometimes, a unit council agenda will change with new information. Then take five or 10 minutes at the end of each unit council meeting to review what was learned, answer questions, and set goals for the next meeting.

47 Build on previously gained knowledge, experiences, and wisdom.

48 Set clear goals with time for feedback in both directions.

49 REMEMBER, EVERYONE HAS A CONTRIBUTION. SOOOOOOOOOOO ...
WHAT ARE YOUR IDEAS FOR SUCCESSFUL SHARED GOVERNANCE?

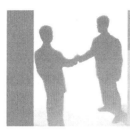

CONCLUSIONS AND RECOMMENDATIONS: WHERE DO WE GO FROM HERE?

After reading this chapter, the participant should be able to:

- State four key messages from the Institute of Medicine and Robert Wood Johnson Foundation Initiative on the Future of Nursing study (2011) for advancing nursing professional practice

- Describe how the recommendations from the Initiative on the *Future of Nursing* study could be supported through shared governance

Why Shared Governance?

> Knowing is not enough; we must apply.
>
> Willing is not enough; we must do.
>
> – *Goethe*

Let's go back for a moment. Where were nurses in 1887?

The following is an excerpt from a job description that was given to floor nurses by a hospital in 1887. It read, In addition to caring for your 50 patients, each nurse will follow these regulations:

- Daily sweep and mop the floors of your ward; dust the patient's furniture and window sills.

- Maintain an even temperature in your ward by bringing in a scuttle of coal for the day's business.

- Light is important to observe the patient's condition. Therefore, each day fill kerosene lamps, clean chimneys, and trim wicks. Wash the windows once per week.

- The nurse's notes are important in aiding the physician's work. Make your pens carefully; you may whittle nibs to your individual taste.

- Each nurse on day duty will report every day at 7 a.m. and leave at 8 p.m. except on the Sabbath on which day you will be off from 12 noon to 2 p.m.

- The nurse who performs her labors and serves her patients and doctors without fault for five years will be given an increase of five cents a day, providing there are no hospital debts outstanding.

Where did nursing go from there?

Over the years, many significant changes occurred to advance nurses and nursing practice to a very different reality today. Nursing became a profession and an interprofessional partner with medicine and pharmacy. Advanced practice nurses, clinical specialists, and nurses with postgraduate degrees in multiple specialties and subspecialties manage their own clinics (nurse practitioners) and work with congregations (parish nurses), criminologists and forensic teams (forensic nurses), and justice departments and attorneys (legal nurse consultants). They are scientists, researchers, and humanitarians. They serve in the military and practice at the bedside, in the home, and in community centers for the homeless and disenfranchised. They are first responders to disasters (hurricanes, floods, and terrorists attacks) and often stay long after others have returned home.

Nurses minister to the physical, emotional, psychological, and spiritual needs of humanity of every age, race and culture, and sociopolitical and economic circumstance according to their own scopes of practice. Many nurses hold advanced degrees at master's, doctoral, and postdoctoral levels. They represent the largest single sector of health professions with more than 3 million registered nurses in the United States today (Institute of Medicine [IOM], 2011).

The job description of 1887 has little to do with this generation of nurses on many fronts. However, there are still such phrases as "other duties as assigned" embedded in job descriptions for nurses at every level of professional and academic preparation and experience, often written by human resources personnel without input from those same nurses. Transactional leaders struggling with staff shortages interpret the phrase "other duties as assigned" to include housekeeping, equipment repair, moving beds, directing traffic (especially around nursing stations), answering phones, and running errands. Without shared governance and collaborative collegiality, nurses cannot engage in the critical duties that affect patient safety, quality of care, and patient outcomes, much less embrace the evolving future of nursing.

Where do we go from here?

Nurse staffing is a matter of major concern because it greatly affects patient safety and quality of care. During a nursing shortage, the delivery of safe, quality patient care can suffer, as the tendency is to create short-term fixes to workforce demands, which ultimately fail to address the real problems. Due to the complex nature and inability to isolate single factors or solutions to this nursing shortage,

  SHARED GOVERNANCE, SECOND EDITION

a systems perspective provides the greatest depth and understanding of the relationship between multiple variables, which incorporate issues in education, health delivery systems and the work environment. Furthermore, the impact of reimbursement, legislation, regulation and technological advances provide for a full appreciation of the nursing workforce shortage complexity. (National League for Nursing, 2001)

Recently, the IOM (2011) put forth dramatic observations and recommendations in their report on the future of nursing. In the opening summary, they lay a strong foundation for implementing shared governance, an organizational management process model, within all levels of professional nursing practice and influence to lead change and advance health:

The United States has the opportunity to transform its healthcare system to provide seamless, affordable, quality care that is accessible to all, patient centered, and evidence based and leads to improved health outcomes. Achieving this transformation will require remodeling many aspects of the healthcare system. This is especially true for the nursing profession, the largest segment of the healthcare workforce. This report offers recommendations that collectively serve as a blueprint to (1) ensure that nurses can practice to the full extent of their education and training, (2) improve nursing education, (3) provide opportunities for nurses to assume leadership positions and to serve as full partners in healthcare redesign and improvement efforts, and (4) improve data collection for workforce planning and policy making. (p. 1)

Based on these observations and the four key messages folded into the proposed blueprint for professional nursing practice, the IOM (2011) reported eight concomitant recommendations:

1. "Remove scope-of-practice barriers. Advanced practice registered nurses should be able to practice to the full extent of their education and training" (p. 9).

2. "Expand opportunities for nurses to lead and diffuse collaborative improvement efforts. Private and public funders, healthcare organizations, nursing education programs, and nursing associations should expand opportunities for nurses to lead and manage collaborative efforts with physicians and other members of the healthcare team to conduct research and to redesign and improve practice environments and health systems" (p. 11).

3. "Implement nurse residency programs. State boards of nursing, accrediting bodies, the federal government, and healthcare organizations should take actions to support nurses' completion of a transition-to-practice program (nurse residency) after they have completed a prelicensure or advanced practice degree program or when they are transitioning into new clinical practice areas" (p. 11).

4. "Increase the proportion of nurses with a baccalaureate degree to 80% by 2020" (p. 12).

5. "Double the number of nurses with a doctorate by 2020" (p. 13).

6. "Ensure that nurses engage in lifelong learning" (p. 13).

7. "Prepare and enable nurses to lead change to advance health. Nurses, nursing education programs, and nursing associations should prepare the nursing workforce to assume leadership positions across all levels, while public, private, and governmental healthcare decision-makers should ensure that leadership positions are available to and filled by nurses" (p. 14).

8. Build an infrastructure for the collection and analysis of interprofessional healthcare workforce data" (p. 14).

In Conclusion

Nurses already provide safe, effective, high-quality, competent care under a plethora of regulatory, business, and organizational conditions and directives. Although the eight recommendations in the IOM report are directed at policymakers, payers, executives, and other professionals from private and public arenas, they resonate with direct-care nurses. The target audience for the IOM recommendations and conclusions may have the power to change healthcare systems nationally and globally; however, the real transformation begins with the nurse engaged in genuine shared governance at the point of service.

Shared governance is the present and future of nursing. Yet implementation of shared governance has made an uneasy journey into professional nursing practice. This work and that of such nurse leaders as Tim Porter-O'Grady, Robert Hess, and Marla Weston (see Appendix 35, expanded bibliography) offer some insight into how to continue to reshape and transform nursing practice:

- When shared governance is newly established (Haag-Heitman & George, 2010; Swihart, 2006)

- When shared governance is in early formations, usually within the first three to five years (Hess, 1998a, 1998b, 2009; Porter-O'Grady, 2004, 2009a, 2009b, 2009c)

- When shared governance is well established, usually after the first five years (Porter-O'Grady, 2004, 2009a, 2009b, 2009c; Weston, 2006)

- When shared governance structures and processes are in trouble (Porter-O'Grady & Basinger, 2010; Porter-O'Grady & Hitchings, 2005; Wright, 2005)

1887 must remain a vague shadow. 2020 beckons. Lived shared governance is professional nursing practice in action. If the IOM recommendations are "building blocks … to expand innovative models of care, … to improve the quality, accessibility, and value of care, through nursing" (2011, p. 278), then shared governance is an organizational management process model that can transform the current culture of healthcare into one that supports and advances those recommendations in diverse practice settings through professional nursing practice. Nurses must drive the future of nursing. Explore the challenges, the possibilities, and the joys that are to come with great purpose and courage. Whatever the future of nursing will be begins now, in the present, with us.

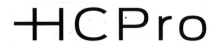